"We all know the difficult decisions and anguish that we go through as loved ones of people with Alzheimer's. Judith London has distilled her years of experience and organized the information in a way that is easy to understand, constructive, and even positive. My mother has been very slowly losing her memory, and through London, I have come to understand that much of my mother's communication difficulties are not only due to her poor memory, but also to her need to receive reassurance that her concerns have been addressed. On Thanksgiving, I instructed my children not to slough off my mother's concerns, but rather to engage her in a conversation about them, answering her questions lovingly and patiently. What a difference this made in enabling my mother to let go of her worries. I highly recommend this guidebook to anyone facing the travails of Alzheimer's. London's guide will be a priceless gift to yourself and you deserve to have it."

—Karen Salzer, Ph.D.

"The radical new frontier of medical science reverses the traditional practice of taking things apart to find out how they work by listening to Aristotle's advice to 'connect the dots.' The whole is more than the sum of the parts. Alzheimer's disease is a summation of multiple vacancies made whole by London's synthesis."

—Walter Bortz, MD, clinical associate professor of medicine at Stanford University School of Medicine and author of *Dare to be 100* and *Longer Living for Dummies*

"London shows us in her book *Connecting the Dots* that what matters most is making a meaningful connection in the moment. Through poignant anecdotes from her clinical experience, she offers us the necessary tools to maintain relationships with our loved ones with Alzheimer's. She inspires us to look beyond the disease and focus on what makes us all the same: our innate longing to be understood and accepted for who we are as well as who we are becoming."

—Janet L. Meiselman, Psy.D., Institute on
Aging in San Francisco, CA

"Reading *Connecting the Dots* brought back many painful memories of my mother, who suffered with Alzheimer's. I would sit with her for hours without finding the appropriate words to comfort her. What a difference it would have made if London's book was available to me at that time. Since my mother loved to dance and this love consumed her after she contracted this disease, I was deeply touched by 'Shall We Dance?,' the beautiful story in chapter one."

—Daniel S. Wilson, Ph.D.

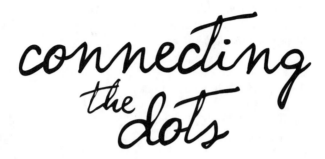

connecting the dots

Breakthroughs in Communication as Alzheimer's Advances

JUDITH L. LONDON, PH.D.

New Harbinger Publications, Inc.

Publisher's Note

This publication is designed to provide accurate and authoritative information in regard to the subject matter covered. It is sold with the understanding that the publisher is not engaged in rendering psychological, financial, legal, or other professional services. If expert assistance or counseling is needed, the services of a competent professional should be sought.

Distributed in Canada by Raincoast Books

Copyright © 2009 by Judith L. London
New Harbinger Publications, Inc.
5674 Shattuck Avenue
Oakland, CA 94609
www.newharbinger.com

FSC
Mixed Sources
Product group from well-managed
forests and other controlled sources

Cert no. SW-COC-002283
www.fsc.org
© 1996 Forest Stewardship Council

Acquired by Melissa Kirk; Cover design by Amy Shoup;
Edited by Kayla Sussell; Text design by Tracy Marie Carlson

Library of Congress Cataloging-in-Publication Data
London, Judith L.
    Connecting the dots : breakthroughs in communication as Alzheimer's advances / Judith L. London ; foreword by Jane E. Brody.
      p. cm.
    Includes bibliographical references.
    ISBN-13: 978-1-57224-502-0 (pbk. : alk. paper)
    ISBN-10: 1-57224-502-6 (pbk. : alk. paper) 1. Alzheimer's disease--Popular works. 2. People with mental disabilities--Means of communication--Popular works. I. Title.
    RC523.2.L66 2009
    616.8'31--dc22

                                                              2009038430

11   10   09

10   9   8   7   6   5   4   3   2   1   First printing

Thank you for understanding that I love you even though I cannot remember your name or exactly who you are.

Thank you for caring for me in such a loving way.

Thank you for reaching out to me, for connecting the dots of what I say, even though I seem like I don't want you to.

What people with advancing
Alzheimer's would say,
if only they could say it.

Contents

PART I
CONNECTING AND COMMUNICATING

CHAPTER 1

CHAPTER 2

CHAPTER 3

PART II
DELVING DEEPER

Acknowledgments

How does one thank all the extraordinary people who provided me with the inspiration, guidance, feedback, and support to make this book a reality?

For starters, my patients with advancing Alzheimer's taught me what I needed to know in order to write this book to tell you that your loved one has plenty to say.

Dr. Frima Christopher taught me that group therapy works for everyone, even those with dementia.

Without the encouragement and mentoring of my good friend Barbara Garshman, former director of development at NBC and a writer herself, I could not have undertaken this project.

My colleague and friend Dr. Kathy Kermit gave me sound professional advice. Joan Anway pointed out pertinent details.

All the people in my writing groups and my instructors, Sylvia Halloran and then Terry Galanoy, supplied valuable feedback. A special thanks to Terry, an accomplished author plus teacher par excellence.

Jan Davis launched me with a publicity piece that led to my finding the wonderful people at New Harbinger, especially my editor, Melissa Kirk, and copy editor, Kayla Sussell.

My family graciously tolerated me, but Bob Davis displayed never-ending patience, listening to me read and reread every one of innumerable versions of the book.

They all made it simple for me.

Foreword

Last winter, as I was dressing after a rejuvenating swim at the YMCA, a woman walked into the locker room looking as if she had just lost her best friend.

In response to my concerned inquiry, she revealed that her mother had Alzheimer's disease and failed to remember—and therefore failed to appreciate—anything her daughter did for her. The daughter felt beaten down by a mix of emotions—anger, frustration, helplessness, depression, and grief—and had no idea how she could continue to cope and communicate with the mother she had once known and loved and now seems to have lost, even though she is still very much alive.

If the daughter had had an opportunity to read the book you now hold in your hands, her emotions and ability to cope with the progressive deterioration of her mother's mental capacity could have been very much improved. In place of helplessness she would have found hope—hope and skills for connecting on a new level with the woman she knew as her mother.

People who have suffered devastating illnesses or injuries are usually faced with the need to adjust to "a new normal." They cannot go back to being the people they once were and must learn new ways to cope with life and find fulfillment. The same is true for their loved ones and caregivers.

Communicating with someone who cannot remember from one minute to the next what has happened or been said can indeed be extremely frustrating and depressing. But the tools described herein can turn frustration into frank enjoyment and illumination. As Dr. Judith London, licensed psychologist, puts it in her introduction, "You can use the tools I acquired from my interactions with my patients to keep communication alive, and to connect, reconnect, and maintain your connection with your loved one."

Years ago I read a most enlightening book: *Ambiguous Loss*, by Pauline Boss, a psychologist at the University of Minnesota. Dr. Boss tells of two sons whose mother had developed Alzheimer's disease. As the disease progressed, the sons continually readjusted the way they communicated with their mother, using humor and fantasy and anything else they could think of to keep the connection alive. By communicating on her level, they maintained a meaningful and enjoyable relationship with their mother, even though she was no longer the woman they once knew.

To be sure, some people, like this woman's sons, have learned these techniques on their own. Most of us, however, could benefit greatly from the professional guidance Dr. London provides. As she puts it, "A connection can arise between people from speaking with each other or from just listening, from hearing music or seeing a beautiful painting together, from reciting poetry or dancing, from singing or praying,...by sitting quietly together or holding hands."

I can see many other uses for the techniques Dr. London describes, from dealing with preverbal children to spending time with someone who is mentally ill, slowed by age, or in the final stages of cancer.

But for people with advanced Alzheimer's disease, the tools Dr. London describes are essential to avoiding resistance, battles, rejection, and a host of other negative reactions that too often are the hallmarks of an uninformed interaction with someone whose sense of reality has been seriously altered. As Dr. London notes, "Those with Alzheimer's have an almost uncanny sense of when someone is being condescending."

In place of condescension, she advocates patience, kindness, consideration, empathy, and a belief that your efforts may pay off. Among her many invaluable guiding principles are these:

- Avoid contradiction and confrontation, which discourage communication and create arguments.

- Remember that a person with Alzheimer's lives in the present, and that each new occasion may require a reconnection—a smile, a warm hello, a reintroduction of who you are.

- Meet the person on his or her own terms.

- Ignore insensitive remarks, respond to them with humor, or say something like "Ouch, that hurts."

From the touching interactions that Dr. London describes, we can more easily keep in mind that while a person with

Alzheimer's may be unable to remember recent events, memories from long ago are the last to be lost. Resurrect them as best you can to keep communication alive: "Remember the time we tried to swim in a glacial lake in Canada and your feet froze in five minutes?" "Remember watching lions mate in Kenya?" Showing pictures can help to stimulate those memories. Consider assembling the most telling photos from the person's life into a small album and look at them and talk about them from time to time.

Try to avoid becoming annoyed when the same question or comment is repeated over and over and over again. Recognize the possibility that incessant repetition may reflect a particular concern or preoccupation and respond accordingly. As Dr. London states, "Repetitive comments can become a springboard for the two of you to interact with each other."

Avoid responding with denial, reason, or logic when confronted with an accusation by someone with Alzheimer's. Instead, take it seriously and apologize, show empathy, or offer to help correct the situation. Many years ago, a neighbor and longtime friend accused my stepmother of taking and not returning her tape recorder. It was laughable on its face, since my stepmother had no use for a tape recorder and had no idea how to work one. But my stepmother was very disturbed by what she viewed as an unjust accusation because she did not know the neighbor's paranoid belief was an early sign of Alzheimer's disease and should not have been taken seriously.

As Americans continue to live longer and longer, thanks to the many tools we now have for preserving good health and modern medicine's ability to patch us up when things go wrong, Alzheimer's disease and other forms of dementia will inevitably visit more and more families. We can all benefit from learning how best to cope with the changes that this disease inflicts upon the mind and emotions of those afflicted and their loved ones. And we can use these techniques in many other aspects of our lives. So, dear reader, read on. You've got nothing to lose and everything to gain by learning how to connect the dots.

—Jane E. Brody, MS
Personal Health columnist for *The New York Times*

Introduction

Wise. Funny. Loving. Insightful. Does this sound like someone you know with advancing Alzheimer's? If not, maybe it's because practically everyone you talk to about Alzheimer's, from professionals to family members, has assumed that once Alzheimer's has progressed and your loved one has stopped initiating conversation, all is lost.

As a psychologist with sixteen years of experience in treating people with advancing Alzheimer's in long-term care settings, I have found this not to be true: you can still reach your loved one. All you need do is to approach the person with Alzheimer's in a caring, responsive way and know how to restore the connection.

That's where you come in. Whether you are a friend, relative, or caregiver of someone with advancing Alzheimer's, this book shows you how to keep communication alive by reaching out and connecting the dots of whatever your loved one says to you. In these pages, you will find the tools you need to communicate and reconnect.

These tools first became apparent to me when I conducted group therapy for advancing Alzheimer's patients. Although group therapy is a popular and effective method for communication and support for people in the early stages of Alzheimer's, this technique is rarely employed when the disease has progressed to the middle and late stages. Those in the early stages who are in support groups claim that the groups are a lifesaver. However, most mental health professionals believe that group therapy cannot benefit people who can no longer remember recent events or learn something new. I believed otherwise.

In order to foster connections and promote communication, once a week for an hour, I met with people who could no longer remember events from day to day or week to week. However, I expected the best from them. The group members rose to the challenge to break through the barriers created by Alzheimer's and communicate. They shared the knowledge that had been locked inside their minds and hearts. We discussed emotional issues, including the hard ones like sadness, frustration, and loss, along with love, compassion, and celebration. Every person in the group made wise and touching comments that inspired me to write this book. Each patient became my teacher. I realized that just because people with advancing Alzheimer's can no longer communicate in their old ways, it doesn't mean that they have nothing to say.

You have known someone living with Alzheimer's and may have been connected to him or her for many years. Or you may be a new caregiver. Whenever you or a few family members meet with your loved one, together you are a group. As a group or as an individual, you can use the tools I acquired from my interactions with my patients to keep communication alive, and to connect, reconnect, and maintain your connection with your loved one.

Part I, chapters 1 through 12, will show you how to go about initiating, connecting, and communicating. Chapter 1 discusses the fundamental nature of connections. Chapter 2 explains how to set the stage so that connecting can take place. Chapter 3 explores the difficulties that can arise when the Alzheimer's patient has problems with hearing and seeing. Subsequent chapters focus on other relevant themes, such as how to handle repetition, dealing with anxiety and depression, and differing communication styles.

Each chapter in part I has a compelling anecdote that displays the uniqueness of these people with advancing Alzheimer's, with the identities of the group members disguised, followed by useful tools revealed in the story. You don't have to know much about the nuts and bolts of Alzheimer's to use the tools. The first six tools form a basis for all connection and communication. The remainder delineates additional ways for you to relate. A summary of the tools appears in the appendix. You can choose the tools that apply to your situation to forge a connection and to communicate.

Part II, chapters 13 through 17, expands your knowledge by providing detailed information on the topics raised in part I, such as providing more information about Alzheimer's and dementia, some good news about Alzheimer's and memory, strategies for coping with difficult behaviors, and taking care of the caregiver: you. A summary of the tools, a glossary of terms, recommended resources, and references can be found in the back of the book.

Note that throughout the book, I intentionally alternate between the pronouns "he" and "she," since the information applies to either gender. And although some of you may be paid caregivers, I refer to the individual with advancing Alzheimer's as "your loved one" as a reminder to the many relatives and friends that someone with this illness is a person with Alzheimer's, not a demented person.

As Alzheimer's advances, your loved one will never be exactly who he was, but you will experience him as he still is: a valuable human being who needs your help to relate to others and to be heard by them. You do not have to accept someone as "gone," when he is very much alive. When you use the tools in this book to reach your loved one and to connect the dots, miracles do happen!

PART I

Connecting and Communicating

CHAPTER 1

Making a Connection:
Shall We Dance?

They were seated in a circle, elderly men and women, the ones who couldn't or wouldn't participate in the exercise or speech programs that day. Not only had their bodies betrayed them, leaving them wheelchair-bound, but their brains had failed them as well. All of them shared a common feature: they were in the middle to advanced stages of Alzheimer's or another form of dementia. They were no longer able to communicate in a conventional way; no longer able to express themselves unless someone prodded them and connected the dots from what they'd said. I was that someone.

I began by asking basic questions: "What is your name? How are you doing today? What's it like for you to not be able to walk?" I directed my questions, one at a time, to each person, coaxing them along, repeating their answers in a loud voice for the hard of hearing. As I went around, one elderly gentleman answered the last question by saying, "I miss dancing. I used to love to dance." A woman across the way chimed in, "So did I!"

And, in the blink of an eye, the man wheeled his chair across the room to that woman. He faced her, stood up from his wheelchair, held out his hands, looked her in the eye, and said, "Shall we dance?" With that, she held up her hands as he reached for them, and they began to sway back and forth, he standing in front of her as she sat. Their faces seemed twenty years younger as they danced to the music that was in their hearts.

. . . .

The look on their faces and their physical touching demonstrated that two individuals can connect beyond words alone. Anything is possible. Who would have thought that a discussion about walking would lead to a dance exhibition? Yet it was a perfect example of the definition of connecting, which is "to bind together; to join." (*Webster's New World College Dictionary*, 3rd ed., 1997). A connection can arise between people from speaking with each other or from just listening, from hearing music or seeing a beautiful painting together, from reciting poetry or dancing, from singing or praying together. It can happen by sitting quietly together or holding hands. Throughout this book, we will be looking at the many ways different ways there are to connect.

The Meaning of Connection

Connecting with each other is a way we share ourselves, one human being with another. This translates into exchanging ideas, laughter, tears, compassion, joy, and sorrow. Our hearts open, and we are filled with elation knowing that someone else understands that special moment as we do. Making a connection creates a bridge so that we are no longer alone. This is a basic human need that continues to exist, even as Alzheimer's progresses.

Quality of the Connection and Alzheimer's

The type of connecting I am speaking of is beyond the simple expression of our mundane but essential needs, such as expressing hunger or thirst. It reaches a higher level where people share emotions and ideas, reveal who they are today, and voice their beliefs. A connection is simply the caring interaction between two individuals so that each senses that the other understands. Make no mistake about this: just because someone is disoriented and confused about day-to-day functions does not mean that her mind is not filled with relevant segments of abstract ideas, opinions, and feelings that she longs to express.

For the person with Alzheimer's, ideas still exist, but the past and present have merged into the same plane. Sentences are made up of pieces of different ideas that don't tie together logically. Many well-meaning relatives and friends just don't take the time to figure out what was said, believing that there is no meaning behind the disjointed phrases. Understandably, a lot of people give up trying to communicate, which leads to a tragic loss of connection when there is still so much to experience together. Any decent quality of life requires us to connect with each other.

The Key

Here is the key: genuine connections follow when you initiate communication and make sense of what your loved one with Alzheimer's is saying. You connect the dots of whatever he says. It isn't mysterious. You simply use the basic tools that I used and connect the remaining "dots" of information your loved one reveals to jump-start the flow of meaningful communication. In that way, you touch the soul within.

When you reach out to restore connections, your loved one with Alzheimer's can connect back with you. The result will be well worth every bit of effort it takes.

CHAPTER 2

Where Do I Start?
Setting the Stage

Kindness. Consideration. Respect. To make connections with your loved one with advancing Alzheimer's, you have to treat her the same way you want to be treated. She is entitled to be regarded as an equal, this individual who had lived a lifetime as an independent, functioning human being long before Alzheimer's began. Treat her with the dignity to which she is entitled. It's hard to let go of preconceived notions that the disease has progressed beyond her ability to relate, but make the leap. Think of her as a person with Alzheimer's, and not just as a demented person. Allow yourself to believe that establishing a connection is still possible, even though she looks withdrawn. In this chapter, we will look at the meaning of communication, and how connecting and communicating begins and then unfolds.

To communicate is defined as "to impart, share, or make common; to pass along, to transmit; to make known; to have a sympathetic and meaningful relationship" (*Webster's New World College Dictionary*, 3rd ed. 1997). Communication is an interactive process and is basic to the way in which we connect. A communication does not have to be intellectual for it to be meaningful. Expressing yourself to another is a complex process, even under ideal circumstances, as we strive to exchange thoughts, opinions, and feelings to create bonds with each other. It is even more of a challenge when Alzheimer's enters the picture to interfere with the transmission of ideas.

Talking is a basic way to communicate. Among couples in which one partner has Alzheimer's, evidence suggests that when the person with Alzheimer's perceives that his partner's words convey respect and caring, are not controlling, and confer dignity upon his remaining competence, the couple's communication improves (Small, Perry, and Lewis 2005). True communication, however, consists of two components: the thought and the feeling. Note that your loved one may be more adept at transmitting a feeling than a thought.

Nonverbal signals such as body language, gestures, facial expressions, and tones of voice complete the communication. The way you speak and the look in your eyes set the stage for connecting to unfold. It all starts with a smile. As someone once said, a smile is the shortest distance between two human beings. Here's how the connection began between one of my "teachers," Susan, and me.

Meet Susan

I entered the unit looking for Susan, whom I had never met. I had reviewed her background and history and I was hoping to engage her in conversation, despite her advancing Alzheimer's dementia. I was also hoping to create a group for group therapy. Susan was the first person I'd considered as a prospective member of the as yet unformed group.

I studied the scene before me: a large room filled with row after row of beds. Faded curtains, currently open, separated the beds. Women seated in armchairs stared vacantly at television sets perched on top of their cluttered bed stands.

As my eyes took in the ward, I saw an elderly person slumped in a wheelchair. I checked the identification number, used to preserve anonymity, above her bed. It matched the number I had obtained. This must be Susan. I moved to her side and sat down on the edge of her bed.

I smiled and said, "Hi Susan. I'm Judy."

No response. I tried again, wondering if she could hear me. I was facing her at an angle, and I lowered my head so she could see me. Then I repeated myself, slowly but loudly. After a long pause, she painstakingly raised her angular, translucent face.

"Hi Susan. How are you doing today?"

Barely audible, she replied, "Not well."

I continued, "Not well physically?" gesturing in a circular fashion to our bodies. No response. "Not well mentally?" gesturing in the same way to our heads.

"Both," she finally replied.

"Ah, that is tough. Does anything hurt?" I asked.

"No," she replied.

"Are you feeling confused?" I asked.

That got her attention. In that moment, when I gave a name to what she was feeling, I think she felt understood.

She peered at me more closely, and I asked her where she was, to continue the exchange. Her clouded blue eyes swept over the open ward scene before her and in a low, uneven voice, she started to tell me what she saw.

"That one over there," she said, pointing to the nurse in charge, "she's the head cook. That one over there," pointing to someone else, "don't ask her for something because she won't give it." I wondered if that person had ever treated her unkindly.

Her voice became stronger. "And all this," she said, moving her arm in a 120-degree arc, "that's where the people come to sit at the tables."

I began to think that she was too impaired to join a group. But as I struggled to make sense of what she was telling me, I suddenly remembered what I had read: for twenty years, Susan had worked as a waitress at a restaurant. She was organizing her surroundings to resemble the dining room of a restaurant, making sense of her confusion.

"This place is a restaurant, isn't it?" I commented, acknowledging her reality.

She smiled at me, a look of relief spreading across her face. I was jubilant. I'd realized that I had just found the first member of my group.

Susan never repeated her conceptualization of the restaurant again, even though we all met in the unit's dining room. Actually, each session began before everyone gathered as a group. I greeted each person individually, introduced myself, and asked her if she would like to join the group that day. When someone was not swayed by my invitation to attend, I respected the occasional, "No, thank you."

To compensate for fleeting memory, I reintroduced myself again when the group had assembled. I made sure that each person had a turn to state her name, and I made sure that I addressed her by name throughout our conversations. One's name represents one's validation as a unique person.

In contrast to many other group members, Susan allowed me to place audio earphones on her ears in order to enhance her hearing ability, and that, of course, helped her to converse. She was a soft-spoken and refined woman. And it turned out that she had a gift for making supportive and loving comments to the others around her.

When she heard someone express herself, Susan would comment, "You are so lovely. You are a wonderful person." When I repeated Susan's comments so that all could hear, appreciation beamed from their delighted faces. Sometimes Susan would reach out her hand to gently touch a person's arm and say, "I love you."

When I was able to piece together her phrases in response to a question, she would light up and say, "You've got it!"

After many months, the staff reported that Susan's physical and mental condition was deteriorating. Despite this, she always attended the group, fully attentive and alert, even when she became so physically and mentally impaired that she had to be transferred to another unit.

One day when we were reintroducing ourselves in the meeting, Susan answered by saying, "You do it for me." I realized that she had forgotten her name, and yet she still felt grateful to be part of the group.

. . . .

Lessons from Susan: Useful Tools and Related Comments

Initially, Susan was slow to respond, a sign of advancing Alzheimer's. I succeeded in starting the connection by placing myself on her level physically, showing her my face, encouraging eye contact, and repeating my greetings. I asked an open-ended question: "How are you doing today?"

Studies show that open-ended questions can produce rich responses from those with Alzheimer's (Small, Perry, and Lewis 2005). There is no right or wrong answer to an open-ended question. Moreover, some research indicates that directly correcting a loved one's response will put an end to the conversation (Gentry and Fisher 2007). I used a yes-no format to check if she was in pain or confused.

To get her attention, I experimented with both verbal and nonverbal communication, including gestures. I approached her with a smile and used short, simple sentences. My tone conveyed friendliness and genuine concern. This is essential because I've discovered that those with Alzheimer's have an almost uncanny sense of when someone is being condescending.

Because I spoke slowly to compensate for the slowdown of her mental processes, Susan had enough time to understand what I said and could respond. The lessons I learned from interacting with Susan revealed some tools that can establish a connection.

Tool 1: Attitude—Treat Your Loved One as a Precious Human Being

- Smile.

- Always introduce yourself and greet your loved one by name every time you meet.

- Position yourself face-to-face or catty-corner on the same physical plane to establish eye contact.

- Use an inviting tone.

- Be kind.

- Be considerate.

- Speak slowly.

- Use gestures as you speak.

- Ask simple but open-ended questions.

- Be patient. Allow time for responses.

- Believe that your efforts may pay off.

I had realized and understood that Susan was confused. Imagine what it must be like to be sitting in unrecognizable surroundings, not knowing where you are, unaware of the time of day, and lost in your own thought fragments. It can be nerve-racking and frightening to be sitting among people you neither know nor recognize. By putting myself into her shoes and guessing that she was confused, I had provided a name for her feeling. When I checked with her, she confirmed my hunch. When I validated her message, Susan sensed that someone had understood her.

Try to picture and feel what your loved one may be experiencing. Have compassion. Take a chance and state what you think she may be trying to say.

Tool 2: Show Empathy

- Put yourself in his shoes to figure out what he may be thinking and feeling.

- Use your intuition about what you think he is saying and feeling. Connect the fragments and see if he agrees.

- Remember that your loved one is a person with dementia, not a demented person.

- Listen.

I didn't expect Susan to formulate such a relatively long response to my question about where she was. Because I reached out and invited her to tell me what she was experiencing, she rose to the occasion and found a way to make sense of her confusion. She demonstrated that she could think, see, and observe, and succeeded in connecting the dots of what she saw around her in light of her earlier experiences.

I would have been completely in the dark about what Susan was communicating had I not familiarized myself with her work history. Having been a waitress for so long, she had organized what she could see of her surroundings into a restaurant configuration and hierarchy, even though she did not consciously remember that she had been a restaurant worker. I had validated her perception and understood it in light of her past.

People with Alzheimer's can organize their confusing world in a logical way based on the mental images that remain. Brain research suggests that memories of a situation or circumstance are experienced as reliving the circumstance in the present moment (Carey 2008a). In that moment, Susan was in a restaurant. By virtue of having shared some history with your loved one, you are in a position to understand what he can recall. He may share something he remembers from his past as if it were happening right now.

If you are a new caregiver, find out as much as you can from friends and relatives who know about the individual, and use the information to relate. Children, grandchildren, daughters-in-law, sons-in-law, nephews, nieces, cousins, and others who help out may not be familiar with past details of the lives of their loved one with Alzheimer's. Learn everything you can to comprehend what she says: where she was born, former jobs, hobbies, and pets. As you try to connect the dots, think back to what you've found out about your loved one's memories from long ago, because the older memories are the last to fade. You may be surprised to discover that in light of knowing more about her, she makes more sense.

Even as your loved one remembers part of her past, she may recall something different in the next moment. Like Susan, she may not refer back to what she said at an earlier time. It may not be on her mind that day.

Keep on trying. Let it flow. Be flexible.

Tool 3: Use What You Know to Go with the Flow

- Use what you know about the person to understand what is being said.

- Acknowledge her reality by repeating her statement back to her and expanding on what she said.

- Go with the flow of your loved one's remarks by following up on what she said.

- Talk about memories from a long time ago since they are the last to fade.

- Don't expect her to remember your previous conversation.

- Remember that she lives in the present moment.

- View each time you meet as an entirely new occasion.

Correcting Susan in any way would have broken the connection. Agreement reinforces the bond. By repeating what she said, you show that you are paying attention. Start off with "As I understand it, you feel that…" and restate what you hear. Contradicting or correcting what your loved one says, especially in a confrontational manner, discourages her from communicating further and undermines her willingness to speak (Gentry and Fisher 2007). Besides, she won't believe you anyway.

Tool 4: Agree

- Don't disagree or argue.

- Acknowledge the thoughts and feelings behind the message.

- Validate what you hear.

Session by session, as the door to communication opened, Susan complimented other group members, told them they were special, and made them feel good about themselves. Every time that she did this, she strengthened her own sense of self. Practically everyone in the group followed Susan's example and expressed support, kindness, and love to each other. In those moments, the feeling of satisfaction radiated from their faces.

Something about being together as a group, week after week, filled Susan and the others with a joy that was reflected in their loving comments to each other. They seemed to know that when they were together, something special was taking place.

After a while, you may notice this happening with your loved one, even when she can't remember exactly who you are.

Tool 5: Have Hope and Express Love

- Express love and support as often as possible and your loved one may reciprocate.

- Focus on what remains, not what is gone.

- Accept her as she is.

The person in your life with advancing Alzheimer's can be your teacher, as Susan was mine. Start by using these tools to connect the dots and rediscover each other.

CHAPTER 3

You Say I'm Shouting? Hearing and Visual Difficulties

Physical changes such as hearing loss and vision problems can interfere with the way a person communicates. Generally, as most people age, they tend to have some trouble with their hearing and vision, whether or not they have Alzheimer's. But these difficulties can be especially troublesome for people with Alzheimer's, who also have difficulty thinking clearly.

Optical conditions, such as cataracts or macular degeneration, also can affect hearing by preventing unconscious lip-reading, which often augments the way someone with a hearing loss "hears" sound. In light of these limitations, caregivers who speak with an accent may be harder to understand. Hearing loss affects any verbal interchange. As you read the anecdote, tools, and related issues in this chapter, you may discover that the manner in which your loved one is affected by hearing loss is an all too familiar story.

It is easier for someone to realize that he isn't seeing clearly than it is for him to admit to himself that he isn't hearing well. He may assume that you are speaking too softly to be heard, and when you raise your voice, you're just too loud. Or when he hears only snippets of what you said, he may guess, inaccurately, and then react to his own misperception. Furthermore, when he cannot hear or clearly see what is going on, he may suspect that people are whispering about him, which leads to feelings of paranoia. The added presence of Alzheimer's makes it even more difficult to communicate because his thinking already has become distorted and his ability to comprehend compromised.

The challenge in communicating with a person with Alzheimer's who also has hearing or vision problems includes adjusting the volume of your voice to be audible, while getting close enough so that he can see your lip movements, yet not so close that he feels threatened. You will see what I mean when you read about Melinda.

Meet Melinda

"She's tiny," was my first thought when I saw her, even though she was sitting perfectly upright in her wheelchair, her straight, white and gray hair cut at chin length, her nose prominent. She reminded me of Miss Haywood, my ballet teacher when I was ten years old. The only thing missing was Miss Haywood's beret.

Melinda was slow to respond to my greetings, even though I was nearly bent in half so that she could see and hear me. I realized she was so hearing impaired that I had to find the balance between raising my voice and coming close to her face, hoping that the cataracts in her eyes would not prevent her from reading my lips.

Suddenly she said in a booming but refined voice, "Don't shout at me!"

I immediately apologized. She looked at me disdainfully. I thought, "There's no way she will ever agree to join a group." However, I knew something about her past life, and I began a conversation.

"What was your profession?" I asked.

She replied regally, "I was a ballerina."

"Where did you dance?"

"I danced for the Royal Danish Ballet," she announced triumphantly. Even late-stage Alzheimer's could not take that away from her.

She ended up joining the group, often making insensitive remarks.

Once when I crouched down to eye level to speak to her to invite her to the group, she proclaimed in a loud voice, "You have bad breath!"

I laughed and replied, "I probably do!" She gave me a wicked grin, and I escorted her down the hall.

The next week, Melinda greeted me with a smile and responded to my usual invitation with "That sounds like a fine idea."

She refused to wear a hearing amplifier, so I decided to wear one as a role model. My strategy failed. So I had to sit next to her to repeat whatever was said directly into her ear. Whenever she spoke, her voice took on a commanding tone. It was easy to imagine her conducting ballet drills after her performance years had ended.

As the months went by, I noticed some changes in Melinda's attitude. I was surprised to see that she had softened. She'd become more aware of the others in the group. After I'd repeated what someone else had said, Melinda began to comment, "That's sad" or "That's a good idea" or "That's right." Her sensitivity to the others also blossomed. One day, as she looked around the group, she spontaneously exclaimed, "That man looks depressed. What's wrong."

I wondered whether she knew that in some way the group was special. I could easily imagine her former ballet students' elation when she said, "Job well done."

. . . .

Lessons from Melinda: Useful Tools and Related Comments

When reading this anecdote, you may have noticed that my approach to Melinda was similar to the one I'd used previously with Susan: be friendly, know the person's background, and integrate this information into conversations to relate to the person with Alzheimer's. I knew two things about Melinda: she was profoundly hard of hearing, and she had been a ballerina. It is very hard to figure out how to project your voice with someone who is hearing impaired. When I spoke too loudly, Melinda chastised me. She never believed that my raised voice was at all related to her hearing deficit.

I never succeeded in convincing Melinda to use an audio amplifier, which is a device to enhance hearing consisting of earphones and a microphone. People with advancing Alzheimer's often view an amplifier with suspicion, not understanding what it is in spite of detailed demonstrations. I resorted to sitting beside Melinda and repeating everything that anyone said so that she could be a part of the conversation. Although this was a cumbersome process, it permitted her to interact with the others.

Nevertheless, even if your loved one refuses to use an amplifier, make the request again a little later, and each time you want to communicate. Don't be discouraged if you continue to be unsuccessful; one time you might just get lucky.

If more than one person is with you when you sit down together, repeat everything that anyone said. Just keep on speaking slowly, face-to-face, to make it easier for your loved one to read your lips while hearing your voice. Try not to yell. Seek a quiet place to sit, with minimal background noise to make it easier for him to hear.

Tool 6: Make Sure You Can Be Heard and Seen

- Always have a hearing amplifier with you, even if your loved one refuses to wear it. An amplifier can be purchased at a general electronics store.

- Reoffer the use of a hearing amplifier each time you want to communicate.

- Be prepared to repeat what you say and, if you are not alone, what others say.

- Place yourself eye to eye so that you can be seen.

By reviewing Melinda's background, as suggested by Tool 3, Use What You Know to Go with the Flow, I knew that she had been a ballerina, and I'd decided to see whether she remembered that part of her past, so that we could establish a connection. Somehow, Melinda had retained the fact that she had been a ballerina. Moreover, she reminded me of my ballet teacher when I was a child. Similarly, you may be reminded of your loved one at an earlier time. You can share what you recall with your loved one by saying, for example, "Grandma, I remember how happy it made me when we took that walk on the beach when I was five."

When Melinda made that uninhibited remark to me about my bad breath, I simply laughed about it, acknowledging her reality. She called things the way she saw them! And she laughed about it too. If that kind of criticism happens to you, don't take it personally. Use humor. Never underestimate the value of laughter to create a connection, even when you might feel insulted.

Tool 7: Don't Take an Unkind Remark Too Seriously

- Have a sense of humor even when insensitive, perhaps even true, remarks are made.

- Try not to take any comment personally, even though it might hurt. If you feel very hurt, let him know simply by saying something like "Ouch. That hurt."

The connection I made with Melinda helped her connect with others. Her social isolation dissolved for that one hour a week. From abrasive, Melinda became supportive, validating the comments that made sense to her. Her gentleness was just behind her cantankerousness; it needed only a little nurturing to reveal itself.

Tool 8: Be Open

- Expect your loved one's mood to change without any warning, and don't be dismayed when this happens.

- Assume he understands, have no expectations that he will respond, and you may be pleasantly surprised.

Ongoing social interaction with your loved one can improve his psychological well-being, as it did for Melinda and others.

CHAPTER 4

But You Just Said That! Beyond Repetition, Repetition, Repetition

Most of us would be surprised to realize how often we repeat ourselves, especially when we are making a point. Repetition is a valuable way to transmit what we know or to learn something new. For an individual with Alzheimer's, repetition is taken to the extreme: she *perseverates*, which is the technical term for the incessant repeating, verbatim, of certain phrases or ideas. Although it can be annoying, it is the only way she may know to communicate, and it can be detrimental to lead her away from the subject. Don't let this discourage you.

Repetition is actually an opportunity for you to connect, and to discover what is beneath the surface of your loved one's mind. Her words tell you what she is thinking, and that is the communication. Experts often advise us to redirect the flow of our words to change the topic or to distract the individual. But that only breaks the connection, diverts your loved one from what she is trying to say, and relieves us, the listeners, of our discomfort.

Instead, think about why your loved one may be repeating that particular idea so that you can explore the subject with her more fully. Use your knowledge about her to figure out why she is repeating herself. Remember that an incessant repetition of the same question or statement reveals a preoccupation or concern with a particular thought in that specific moment.

Here is a story about Donna, whose repetitive statements of various subjects became an opportunity for me to discover what was on her mind. Eventually, those statements became the springboard for connecting and communicating more deeply.

Meet Donna

"I like the baked potato, the jacket potato, coleslaw, and juice. No smokin', no drinkin', no alcohol." Donna, a stout woman with white hair, spoke firmly, her voice lilting along, the speed of her speech like the click, click of high-heeled shoes on a wooden floor. As soon as she had completed this recitation, within minutes she would begin it again, repeating the identical words.

I thought to myself, "This is a perfect example of perseveration." I wondered how to respond before she began again.

"Donna, you have an amazing memory for these things," I commented, hoping she would explain her remarks more fully.

In response, she grinned broadly and said, "My mother always told me, 'Never throw food away; give it away.'"

By then, I realized that I must respond quickly about what she had said before she could repeat yet another set of facts imprinted on her brain. "Tell us more about your mother," I said, hoping she would delve deeper so I could involve the others in a discussion about their mothers. It worked! Donna reported that her mother had been a nurse. She even listened for a while as others spoke. This was progress.

However, Donna soon interjected, "Did you know that there were 65 million people in California, 30 million cars, and it costs five dollars for a cup of coffee in Paris?"

"Where did she get this information," I wondered, these clusters of unrelated facts that regularly flashed through her brain and were repeated time after time? I asked her, "You know so many facts, Donna. Where did you learn them all?"

"I once heard Dianne Feinstein, the mayor of San Francisco, speak and that's what she said. Fine woman, that Dianne Feinstein," she added. That explanation helped me understand that someone whom Donna had admired had inspired her to remember these "facts."

Donna infused the group with her energy. Every time she repeated one of her fact-filled statements, the topic was established for that part of the session, and I explored the ideas that lay beneath the surface of what she said. It became a routine. Most group meetings started with a discussion of the members' favorite foods, then moved on to the plight of going hungry, lessons from our mothers, and commentary on how expensive things were. Donna had become the informal discussion leader, and by my searching deeper, she elaborated on her opinions. One day when the subject of food arose again, I asked, "How do you know so much about food, Donna?"

"I used to work at a cafeteria that served great food." When prodded, she added, "I always gave the homeless men food when they came to the side door. Didn't want them to go away hungry."

"What a lovely way to show you cared."

Donna nodded her head in agreement.

In a discussion about dance, Donna told us that she'd loved to go dancing in the city's major ballrooms. Another group member chimed in that he had loved to dance and romance the ladies, before his debilitating stroke. By reminiscing about their good times, they both connected and relived experiences from which they'd had much pleasure.

Donna was also a master card player. She loved to play Kings in the Corner, a card game I didn't even know. (It was probably just as well, since it was rumored that she made up her own rules.) She always had a deck of cards in her pocket, only she never remembered that they were there. "Hey," she'd call out, "Somebody stole my cards!"

Nurses aides would come to her and say, "Look in your pocket, Donna."

She'd look, and she'd become so happy and surprised to find them.

I always served ice cream to the group, knowing the importance of sensory stimulation. Ice cream was a treat that invoked a memory of its own; it became the stimulus for discussions of past celebrations. Donna always exclaimed that she loved eating it.

One day, out of the blue, Donna asked, "What is the name of this group?" She had moved beyond repetitive statements into asking a question; one based on a more abstract idea. It was a major advance. When Donna wondered whether the group had a name, that showed she understood where she was at that moment.

I replied, "Let's talk about that. What do you think we should call it?" Everyone listened, expectantly.

"I think we should call it 'The Ice Cream Group,'" Donna said.

"What do you think of that name?" I said to the others.

"I think it's a great name," a participant responded. And so it was.

Amazingly, Donna remembered the group name most weeks, perhaps because her preoccupation with food and her delight in eating ice cream had inspired her to think of a name for the group in the first place.

The first time I heard Donna say, after two spoonfuls of ice cream, "I've had enough. Give it to the hungry people," was a sad day for me. Her lack of interest in eating ice cream made me realize that she was entering the final phase of Alzheimer's.

Donna had fought the good fight.

. . . .

Lessons from Donna: Useful Tools and Related Comments

Donna was a lively woman with an outgoing personality and a great concern for others. I saw her repetitious speech as an opportunity to connect and communicate with her, because I realized that her repetitions were her way of connecting and communicating with me and others.

Looking back at the beginning of our interactions, I used Tool 3, Use What You Know to Go with the Flow, which acknowledged her reality. That helped me to connect with Donna. Asking her about her interest in food created a pathway for her to think a little more, and for me to pick up on what she was saying. Repetition was her form of communicating with others, revealing what was on her mind.

When she continuously repeated herself, staff and visitors often tried to distract her. Before I discovered the source of her constant repetitions, no one had had any idea that there might be some meaning attached to her incessantly repeated statistics. When directed to dig a little deeper, Donna reached the next level of thought, and she appreciated being heard.

When your loved one keeps saying the same things over and over, redirect the subject back. For example, when Donna mentioned her mother, I asked her to say more about her, to validate whatever she might say. Keep inviting your loved one into the conversation, keep asking for his input. Expand on his comments by adding on what you think, as recommended in Tool 3.

For example, I was floored when Donna spontaneously asked about the name of the group, never expecting her to think about it. I redirected the question back to the entire group, realizing that she'd had an idea to share and she, appropriately, named it The Ice Cream Group. Not only had Donna made a connection between a pleasurable oral sensation and the group itself, but she had initiated the idea on her own. Often, listening and responding to the content and feelings behind your loved one's statements will break the chatter, help you understand why the subject is so important, and validate the message that what she is saying is worthwhile. In that way, your loved one's repetitive comments can become a springboard for the two of you to interact with each other.

Tool 9: Use Your Loved One's Repetitions to Connect

- Constant repetition is an opportunity to communicate.

- Delve beneath the statements to find meaning.

- Ask your loved one for her opinion about any issue that is brought up.

- Connect the fragments to help her express herself.

When an object is out of sight, many people with Alzheimer's cannot figure out where it might be. So they often accuse others of stealing their property. Friends, relatives, and caregivers find these allegations hard to deal with and may take them personally, which leaves them feeling insulted and angry. Such accusations may also be a sign of mild paranoia, not uncommon in Alzheimer's, given the random pattern of brain cell damage, especially if compounded by hearing loss. For more on paranoia, see chapter 9.

Whenever Donna forgot where she had put her playing cards, she accused others of stealing them. If your loved one, like Donna, makes such accusations, reason and logic are usually futile. The best way to deal with the allegation is to take her seriously. Acknowledge her perception by saying, "You think that I took... That's upsetting. Let me help you find it," and defuse the situation. Help locate the misplaced item together. As recommended in Tool 2, show empathy about what it's like to lose something you value, whether or not there are grounds for your loved one's contention. If she suspects you of doing something wrong, apologize by saying, "I'm so sorry if I upset you. I didn't mean to."

Tool 10: Deal with Accusations

- Acknowledge that an item is not there or validate your loved one's perception that something is wrong. Be sympathetic.

- Offer to help him find what is missing or to straighten out the situation.

- Apologize if your loved one says that you did something wrong.

- Once again, don't take it personally.

To stimulate pleasant sensations and recollections that you both can share, talk about some of your loved one's favorite foods or socially significant foods, such as ice cream, hot chocolate, or coffee. Avoid talking about or offering alcohol because it contributes to unsteadiness, confusion, and forgetfulness. Your loved one may astonish you with some new reminiscences.

Tool 11: Use Foods to Awaken Memory

- Offer your loved one a favorite food or nonalcoholic drink.

- Use food as a springboard to awaken memory and pleasant sensations.

Typically, a lack of interest in eating any food, especially favorite foods that have previously brought delight, is a signal that the long battle with Alzheimer's is nearing its end. More information about the last phase of Alzheimer's will be found in chapter 13.

CHAPTER 5

Did You Hear the One About...? Styles of Communication

There are so many ways that people talk to each other, often alternating between one approach and another. For example, your speech style can depend on whether you are speaking to a dear friend or a salesperson. Individuals even speak differently to the same people in different situations. Each person has his own style of communicating. Even repetition can be considered a speech style. Some people talk a lot, while others are basically quiet. Creative expression through photography or art is a powerful nonverbal method of communication. In addition, men and women may have entirely different patterns of communication.

As Deborah Tannen (1990) pointed out, most men tend to connect by communicating facts, figures, stories, and jokes to establish their status or independence and to make them feel noticed and respected. Most women tend to converse by sharing feelings and experiences, which usually results in connection and intimacy. Of course there are always exceptions, as we saw with Donna. When recent facts and figures are no longer recalled and it is harder to remember one's past achievements with no new ones to report, men, in particular, can be at a loss for something to say.

Women, in general, tend to be more open about revealing their feelings, whereas men may minimize their feelings to maintain their masculine image of themselves. As a rule, men use factual information to initiate bonds with each other. Jimmy, however, was a man with advancing Alzheimer's who used many ways to communicate.

Meet Jimmy

When I would stop by to see Jimmy, he was usually lying down on his bed, fully clothed, eyes half closed. Sometimes he would refuse my invitation to join in the group by saying, "I'm not feeling well." After extending my sympathies, I'd reluctantly walk away, and within minutes he'd be up and following me, his energy returning.

Jimmy was one of the lucky ones. He was eighty years old and still able to walk, and when he did, he bounced up and down as he strode along with his walking cane. He spoke in short, clipped sentences, and there wasn't much depth in what he said, but each sentence was a complete thought that revealed what was actually on his mind. Once engaged, he smiled easily and often.

Jimmy loved football and wearing his New York Giants hat, but his favorite person in the world was his mother. A photo of a young dark-haired beauty, his mother in her youth, was always on his night table and a photo of a gray-haired elderly woman, his mother in her later years, was tacked to the wall of his room.

"Have I shown you this picture of my Mom?" he would ask, and I would always say no, even though he had shown the picture to me innumerable times. "I wish you could have known my Mom," he continued, "I miss her more and more every day. After she fell down and broke her hip, she went into a nursing home. She got Alzheimer's," Jimmy said, apparently unaware that he had this disease, too.

As for the Giants, he commented, "I had season tickets to every one of their home games since 1947."

Like many others with Alzheimer's, he would repeat these things every time I, or anyone else for that matter, saw him. But no one minded; he was such a well-mannered and polite fellow. He also loved telling slightly off-color jokes. "Do you know who is sleeping with cats?" he'd ask.

"No," I replied, although I had heard him tell this joke many times.

"Mrs. Katz!" he'd answer, grinning from ear to ear as he watched me laugh.

Jimmy remembered that when he was working, he had traveled around town by public bus. He also told me about the attractive woman he had met while going to work, and, wistfully, how much he wished that she hadn't moved away. But they had been only "bus" buddies, because Jimmy had never been able to muster up the courage to ask her out on a date.

One day, he handed me a drawing of a man's head in profile. The strokes were clean and well-defined, but the man's forehead protruded slightly from the face. "Here, I want you to have this," he said, as he presented it to me. I was surprised.

"Why, thank you, Jimmy. Who is this?" I asked.

"Me," he answered, with a crooked grin.

"I will treasure it, Jimmy."

I went back to my office and placed Jimmy's self-portrait on the wall directly above my desk in the place of honor it deserved.

· ·

Lessons from Jimmy: Useful Tools and Related Comments

Using a positive and empathic tone, as suggested in Tool 1, Treat Your Loved One as a Precious Human Being, and Tool 2, Show Empathy, helped me to connect with Jimmy. When he realized that I had acknowledged what he'd said, he mustered up the energy to attend. Many people need encouragement to participate in an activity, including a conversation, and people with Alzheimer's need even more encouragement, because of their problems with initiating any activity.

I learned a lot about football and baseball when I met with men like Jimmy. He exemplified the way in which men tend to relate by talking about sports and current events and telling jokes. Every session, I'd ask Jimmy how the New York Giants were doing, and he would regale me with their triumphs and sorrows. Other men in the group added fragments of news events to the group conversation, and we discussed their thoughts and reactions to these bits of news.

Jimmy delighted in telling jokes—the three that he remembered. Nevertheless, everyone laughed at the jokes' endings despite the countless times he had told them. Many men enjoy telling jokes. Laughter is a heartwarming affirmation. Usually, women express humor in a different way, such as by sharing a common, funny experience. Either way, laughter is good for the soul and encouraging it produces a connection.

Tool 12: Some Openers to Use with Men

- Introduce news about sports or other current events as a way to communicate.

- Again, restate what you hear.

- Listen to a joke and laugh, no matter how many times you've heard it.

- A sense of humor endures for a long time. Have fun laughing together.

As Jimmy perseverated, or repeated himself, which was one of the ways he could relate to others, he introduced themes important to others in the group, such as dealing with loss. For example, Jimmy remembered his mother. His answers to open-ended questions helped him to delve beneath his recurring statements about her and allowed him to mourn her passing. Talking about her gave others permission to speak of those they'd lost too. Because of his mother's pictures and his preoccupation with her, Jimmy introduced the theme of loss week after week. Many other groups that met on different units also gravitated to discussions on loss, a theme addressed in detail in chapter 6. When a person with advancing Alzheimer's speaks about the passing of a significant person or, for that matter, of any loss, encourage him to say more. It will promote healing.

Tool 13: Acknowledge Loss

- Acknowledge and discuss any kind of loss.

- Talk about your loved one's parents or other beloved family members to stimulate conversation and promote healing. Ask questions like "What was your mother like?"

- Acknowledge and explore feelings, even the sad ones, whether or not he realizes that the relative is gone.

A photograph of a person can stimulate a meaningful interaction with a loved one who, like Jimmy, can still initiate a conversation. Keep photographs of the important people or events in your loved one's life and assemble them into a small album, perhaps with your loved one helping out. If he does not initially respond to your effort to verbally interact, you can take out the album to relate and say, "Let's look at some pictures. We all had such a good time at that party. Look at you. You have such a big grin on your face."

Tool 14: Use Meaningful Photographs to Relate

- Use photographs and make comments to stimulate memory and to relate.

- Say something about the photograph.

- Explore your loved one's response.

Making art together is a valuable way to communicate and connect. Creating or viewing art projects with each other can be an opportunity for self-expression and connection. Many people with advancing Alzheimer's and other dementias have astonished us with their artistic ability and interpretations of various works of art. In an article in the *New York Times*, it was reported that people with early Alzheimer's actively participated in discussions about fine art paintings when on an outing to a museum (Kennedy 2005). As Alzheimer's advances, making paintings may continue to stimulate self-expression.

Jimmy's self-portrait was a remarkable likeness, except for the protruding forehead. In drawings made by someone with Alzheimer's, facial distortions and other misrepresentations may reflect the changes in visual perception that the disease produces. Nevertheless, painting, drawing, collaging, and working with clay are all wonderful vehicles for nonverbal self-expression and the chance to interact.

Jimmy's message to me was clear: he wanted me to have the sketch, which was a concrete symbol of our connection, because he wanted me to remember him.

Tool 15: Use Art as a Way to Relate

- Create art with your loved one to inspire self-expression and connection.

- Discuss the meaning of what you both produce.

- Elicit your loved one's opinion about a painting you both view and ask, "What do you think of it?" Or you can ask, "What do you think it is saying?"

In light of your shared history together, you may want to devise your own creative methods to connect with your loved one.

CHAPTER 6

What Have I Lost? More About Loss and Forgetfulness

Your loved one with Alzheimer's faces the loss of some of the most basic aspects of an adult's life: being independent; having a career; engaging in personal interests; taking care of himself and his bodily functions; thinking clearly; understanding others' speech; speaking coherently; and of course, initiating communication. And he knows that he cannot remember. Forgetfulness is an ever-present loss. In addition, he is losing the ability to participate in relationships as a trusted partner, parent, or friend. You are suffering from that loss as well.

Further loss lies in the changes he experiences from whom he used to be. When someone's ability to function or to express himself deteriorates, his self-esteem diminishes. *Self-esteem* is your belief in yourself, your self-respect, and being proud of who you are. Being able to reach out to people reaffirms your sense of self, whereas not being able to initiate contact diminishes your sense of self. Your loved one may be struggling to preserve his sense of self (Holst and Hallberg 2003).

Loss occurs throughout one's lifetime, Alzheimer's notwithstanding. Talking about who and what we no longer have, including the death of a loved one, gives us the opportunity to come to terms with our sorrow. In one study, 92 percent of those with dementia spoke of the impact of the losses they had sustained (Ostwald, Duggleby, and Hepburn 2002). The participants in the groups I led, despite the advance of the disease, still had plenty to say about losing their parents, pets, homes, independence, and memory.

Here are two reactions to loss and forgetfulness, the first from Iris, who brought loss one step further, followed by Lee.

Meet Iris

"Equal rights for women! Equal rights for women!" Iris had been an ardent feminist, a firebrand of a woman, and an activist throughout her life. Now she sat before me in a wheelchair, her hair pure white, still thick, and cropped short. Her eyes were flashing, her voice was deep and resonant, and she sang Broadway tunes with vitality. When Iris belted out "Oh, What a Beautiful Morning," everyone joined in, including me. We sounded like a community chorus! And when she resumed singing it later on, right in the middle of a discussion, everyone stopped and sang once again.

But when Iris stopped singing and opened her mouth to speak, the few words she said made no sense. "What is that definition of a sentence that I learned in elementary school?"

I asked myself. My memory kicked in and I remembered: "A sentence is a group of words expressing a complete thought." Iris's words were there, but they were scrambled into fragments. It was hard to piece the fragments together to form complete thoughts. When I got it right, she would say, "Exactly!" If I was off the mark, she'd let me know that too, by saying no and shaking her head from side to side.

In the group, someone mentioned the death of a loved one, which lead to a discussion about loss. As we went around the room, I asked each person if she had ever lost anyone or anything. People spoke of their mothers, about their pets that had died, and about missing their homes, their independence, and their memory.

When it was Iris's turn and I asked her if she'd ever lost anything, she paused and thought about my question. Then she declared, "Yes!"

And when I asked her what she had lost, she replied simply, "Myself." And so, she had.

Struck by her comment, I said, "That must be so hard." She remained silent.

I told Iris that we knew she was still there, and that she was great at remembering and singing songs. She gave me a quizzical smile, not really believing what I said.

· ·

Lessons from Iris: Useful Tools and Related Comments

Alzheimer's can strike anyone, regardless of her station in life. Iris had been a political activist. Apparently, some of her oratorical skills had remained, judging from the way that she could project her voice, but too many connections had been broken for her to make much sense.

Singing gave Iris a way to express herself and to connect with others. Music is a powerful tool for jogging the long-term memory, as you will see in chapter 7. Most of the time, Iris was able to remember the words to the songs she sang. As the disease progressed, she could hum only the melodies. Iris's singing brought everyone together. When others joined her, each one would bask in the joy of sharing the experience. When her singing interrupted conversations, I had to sing along and use Tool 3, Use What You Know to Go with the Flow.

Tool 16: Use Singing and Music to Connect

- Music is a wonderful way to cross the barriers of isolation.

- Music can communicate beyond words alone.

- Be courageous and sing along. It's fun!

Iris spoke in an almost incomprehensible way. Your loved one may do the same some of the time. Keep on connecting the dots of the words or phrases that she says. You can be sure that she will tell you if you have accurately articulated her sentiments, as Iris told me. Keep on using Tool 3 and go with the flow.

Even though Iris used nearly the same words heard by Dr. Alois Alzheimer (for whom this disease is named) in 1906, when his patient Auguste D. stated, "I have lost myself," I was not prepared to hear Iris say it. We can only imagine how dispiriting and tragic it is to lose oneself, one's identity, one's very essence. And Iris, like Auguste D., knew that, indeed, she had lost herself.

At some point, your loved one may say to you that she has lost herself. As heartbreaking as it is for you to hear this, offer comfort and tell her how much she still means to you. Remember Tool 13, Acknowledge Loss, and acknowledge her loss and be compassionate, even as your heart aches.

I told Iris that she had made an important contribution to the group anyway. But she remained unconvinced.

Meet Lee

As Lee sat in a wheelchair, her snow-white, wavy hair framing her wrinkled but still patrician face, her brow was furrowed. She looked puzzled as I approached her. I brought my face closer to hers, knowing that was the best way I could count on her recognizing me because of her blurred vision and loss of hearing.

"Hi, I'm Judy," I said. "We would love to have you join us in our weekly discussion group."

She looked at me with no sign of recognition, although she had been attending the group for over four years. Reluctantly, she replied in a resigned voice, "I guess I'll go because you are telling me to."

"You don't have to go if you don't want to. But, what else do you have to do?"

She hesitated a minute, then answered, "I'll go."

I moved her wheelchair away from her bed, steered her down the hallway, turned left into the "group" room, which was actually the dining room with the tables and chairs pushed back to the walls, and wheeled her inside, positioning her at the far end of the room to allow space for the others.

"I'll be back in a few minutes," I said, this time speaking close to her right ear where I knew that some hearing remained. When I returned, I placed people on either side of her. Gradually, she raised her head, her eyes vacant, glanced to one side and then the other, and slowly a look of recognition spread across her features. Her eyes sparkled as if a lightbulb had been turned on.

"I know," she exclaimed, with an animated voice, "I'm here with my friends." Her face grew radiant as the others arrived.

Lee often told the people in the group how much she loved them. These proclamations of love were a sharp contrast to the way she spoke to some of her relatives and caregivers, for whom she often expressed grouchiness. But something came over Lee when we all met together. She would say that she felt great that day because "all the people I love are in this room."

When the group members talked about how to cope with life, Lee said, "I pray to God that I will be all right. And then, when I wake up the next day, I thank God that I am still alive." From time to time, Lee would quietly note, "I wish God would take me now."

Once we were all talking about aging and getting old, and Lee said, with a knowing smile, "I am very old. It's just fine." When I escorted her back to her area after the session ended, she suddenly said, "Getting old is shitty!" We both laughed.

At another meeting I asked each person how she felt about her problems with remembering. One person stated, "It makes me cry and cry."

Then Lee chimed in with this statement: "Now that I'm *non compos mentis*, I'm glad that I have forgotten a lot of the unhappy things from my life."

Then she grinned her cheerful grin, from ear to ear.

· ·

Lessons from Lee: Useful Tools and Relevant Comments

Lee did not remember the group or know who I was when she saw me out of context. This can happen to anyone. You can see people who look familiar, but you cannot place them because you associate them with the context in which you know them. For example, you might not remember the person who was riding the stationary bike next to you in the gym this morning when you meet her in the grocery store. I didn't get upset that Lee had forgotten me, but if she had been my mother, it would have stung.

Lee didn't recall anything about the group until the people with whom she usually met arrived and they were seated in a familiar arrangement. Then she made the connection, to her utter delight.

**Tool 17: Set Up the Same Seating Location
to Jog Memory**

- Establish a regular seating arrangement each
  time you sit down to relate.

- Using the same configuration may improve
  your loved one's ability to recognize people and
  places.

One of the ways that Lee coped with the difficulties in
her life was to pray. Prayer and spirituality play a significant
role for many others too. (See chapter 7 for a discussion of
how prayer can help those with Alzheimer's.) Lee was tired
and probably depressed when she made the comment about
being old, and she wished that "God would take me now."
When she was not feeling tired or depressed, her attitude
was more in line with her statement, "I'm glad that I have
forgotten a lot of the unhappy things from my life."

As you undoubtedly know, a person can feel happy one
moment and sad the next. In fact, it appears that there are
many areas of the brain that govern emotion, and one of
these is the last to be affected by Alzheimer's, as you will see
in chapter 14.

The capacity to love and to be loving survives despite
Alzheimer's. Love is not forgotten. Lee might not have remembered a name, but she knew those she liked and loved, and
she let them know. Tool 5, Have Hope and Express Love,
reminds us to have hope and not to forget about expressing
our love. As Alzheimer's advances, feelings can persist for a
long time.

Your loved one wants you to reach out so that she can express her love. Use Tool 2, Show Empathy. Just keep on listening and responding.

When looking at memory loss, most people assume that losing one's memory has no benefits whatsoever, especially when certain memories were a source of comfort. For Lee, however, forgetting served to erase the pain of some past unhappy experiences. And she was able to state her opinion with a power of speech no one had ever heard from her before. Lee was eloquent.

CHAPTER 7

Who Can I Turn To? Prayer, Song, and Spiritual Connection

Prayer, song, and spiritual connection are interrelated. *Prayer* may be defined as an earnest, sincere, humble request, a spiritual communication with a higher power. According to *Webster's New World College Dictionary* (1997) to pray means "to ask very earnestly; to make supplication." *Spiritual* refers to a life-giving force, as of the spirit or the soul, as distinguished from the corporeal or the body. Thus the act of praying is a communication that transcends the physical, materialist world. An individual may go to a house of worship to pray with other people as a community. Or a person can engage in personal prayer in solitude and communicate directly with her higher power in her own fashion. For those who believe in the power of prayer, praying can ease their burdens and uplift their souls.

People often learn the ritual of prayer at an early age. When a person with Alzheimer's has a history of engaging in prayer, she maintains her ability to pray even as the disease progresses. People like Lee and others receive solace from praying. Your loved one may be someone who remembers prayer. She may find that praying comforts her, offering her reassurance that a higher power will take care of her during this confusing and frightening time in her life. If you are a family member, friend, or caregiver of someone with Alzheimer's, prayer may serve the same function for you. If you have faith, you may find in prayer some consolation that you are not alone during this challenging time.

A spiritual connection can be maintained with or without a religious practice. An article in *American Family Physician* (Anandarajah and Hight 2001) describes spirituality in terms of finding meaning, hope, comfort, and a sense of inner peace. Given this explanation, the possible paths you can follow to experience spirituality expand to incorporate music, singing, laughter, art, poetry, nature, and meditation.

Dr. Joan Borysenko (2008) emphasizes that love is an indispensable component of spirituality. Sharing any experience can produce a sense of belonging and become a means to uplift your spirits, restore hope, and establish a connection. An activity that brings about a spiritual bond can bring healing to the soul.

Many spiritual approaches endorse learning how to live in the present moment as one of the highest manifestations of human spirituality. Alzheimer's, by its very nature, induces a situation in which a person lives primarily in the present, even as past memories merge with current awareness. *Ironically, it appears that, as the disease advances, your loved one with Alzheimer's achieves one of the highest forms of spiritual enlightenment by living in the moment.*

Music and singing can reach your loved one when other approaches may not. Listening to or singing melodies may be the way that she can connect with her past, connect with others, or offer her a way to express religious exaltation. However it functions, music touches everyone's essence. Research supports the value of music, linking listening to music with increased relaxation and finding that this response generally appears to be unaffected by Alzheimer's disease (*American Journal of Alzheimer's Disease and Other Dementias* 2006). Meaningful exchanges with a loved one may foster spiritual connection. Singing with each other or listening to music that you know your loved one used to enjoy can lift the two of you to a heartwarming place for that moment, as you will soon see with Agnes.

Meet Agnes

Agnes sat with her eyes hidden behind oversized glasses; her graying light-brown hair was frizzy and had tendrils falling on her thin-skinned, freckled face. A devout Catholic her entire life, whenever we talked about how to cope with feeling sad or forgetful, Agnes would say in that sing-song, shaky voice of hers, "I pray." Other group members would nod in agreement.

After some of the others shared the information that they prayed, Agnes would tentatively start singing "Amazing Grace," her voice growing stronger as she sang. She often missed some of the words but never wavered from the melody. Everyone joined in. She still had a beautiful voice, well schooled from her years of singing in her church choir. Singing hymns and praying often occurred during group sessions. Sometimes we were regaled with Christmas carols, even in the middle of August.

Despite her memory loss, Agnes knew when people were repeating the same story week after week, and she would say, "Oh, no. Not that again. We heard that already!" although she herself would do the same thing.

I realized that it would do little good to point out that her remark hurt someone else's feelings, so I responded by saying, "People repeat themselves because that's what's on their minds, and they just can't stop saying it over and over again." She looked at me with a silent "harrumph" and soon forgot the subject, until it happened again.

In the unit, Agnes was often concerned about the woman in the bed next to hers. Agnes often inquired about her health and called her a friend. She frequently said, "I love you," to the woman. But one day, Agnes turned against her and no one could figure out why. Agnes began to make mean comments like, "You're ugly. I don't like you."

The woman in the next bed was crushed, hurt by what Agnes said. No matter what we did or said, Agnes would not budge; her roommate continued hurting until we moved her away.

Prayer and music never changed Agnes's mind.

. . . .

Lessons from Agnes and Related Comments

Regardless of the progression of the disease, the ability to pray remained intact for Agnes, who had prayed often in the past. She had strong religious conviction, which she joyously expressed by singing hymns. Others followed her lead, especially when she sang "Amazing Grace," a hymn so popular that she and the others still remembered it, bringing comfort to them all. Agnes succeeded in forming a connection by singing, further reinforcing how Tool 16, Use Singing and Music to Connect, can work. Prayer played a powerful role in Agnes's ability to cope and survive.

Tool 18: Use Prayer if It's Appropriate

- Prayer can be a healing experience. Acknowledge prayer.

- Use prayer if it's appropriate for you or your loved one.

- Living in the moment is the reality for you and your loved one.

Agnes's faith and her behavior were often at odds with each other. Among other things, Agnes could not tolerate other people repeating themselves. In this case, I chose not to confront her directly, remembering Tool 3, Use What You Know to Go with the Flow. I knew that her mind was too rigid to be able to think about someone else's feelings when she was focusing on what was bothering her, but I provided an explanation for the others' benefit. And in the next minute or two, Agnes forgot about her annoyance and moved on.

There was no discernable event or apparent reason to account for Agnes's about-face toward the woman in the bed next to hers. Sometimes people with Alzheimer's suddenly turn on someone whom they have loved. There is so much we don't understand about the manifestations of the erratic destruction of brain cells. Internal cues, biochemical changes, or neural breakdowns can trigger unanticipated behavior. When that occurs, nothing can penetrate the new mind-set. In Agnes's case, at least, we were able to alter the environment by moving her former friend to another place in the unit.

If your loved one suddenly launches a verbal attack, the guideline is don't take it personally, a recommendation pinpointed in Tool 7, Don't Take an Unkind Remark Too Seriously. You have an advantage that Agnes's friend did not: you can grasp the idea that your loved one may be reacting to a stimulus that has nothing to do with you. Of course, it hurts anyway. Nevertheless, you have an obligation to yourself to process your feelings with someone who can understand all of the issues involved. (See chapter 16 for more information.) It is futile to do that with your loved one, who will neither believe you nor remember that she has made unkind remarks.

Tool 19: There's Not Always a Simple Answer for a Change in Attitude

- Your loved one may make mean remarks.

- You can't expect your loved one to be reasonable.

- Accept her limitations.

- Your loved one may not respond to any approach.

- No one has all the answers for someone's behavior.

- Change the environment since your loved one cannot change.

- Don't take it personally.

- Find support from others who know what it's like and share your feelings.

People with Alzheimer's experience mixtures of contrasting mental states, as seen with Agnes. Living in the moment also implies that your loved one may be unable to extend a spiritual connection from one circumstance to another. Nonetheless, you still can be part of creating a spiritual bond, whatever the path.

CHAPTER 8

I Feel So Troubled: Anxiety and Depression

When you think about it, you can see why someone with dementia could be uneasy and unable to say so due to his impaired ability to communicate. Your loved one can't talk about how he feels, so he acts out with symptoms such as restlessness, persistent irritability, apprehension, sleep disorders, loss of appetite, withdrawal, shouting, or even physically striking out at others.

Statistics on the prevalence of anxiety in people with Alzheimer's vary from 25 percent to 60 percent. One study found that 70 percent of the participants exhibited symptoms of anxiety (Teri et al. 1999). The conditions of anxiety and depression are related: someone who is nervous may become overwhelmed with sadness, tearfulness, or thoughts of suicide, and someone whose mood is basically sad may become jittery. The overlap between these two conditions may be as great as 54 percent (Teri et al. 1999).

You, as a caregiver of a person with Alzheimer's, may also experience anxious feelings or gloominess when you contemplate how your life has changed because of the disease. The many issues you face as a caregiver are addressed in depth in chapter 16.

The rate of depression among people with Alzheimer's averages 30 percent, with some studies reporting rates as high as 87 percent (Teri et al. 1999). A person may become disheartened on first learning of the diagnosis of Alzheimer's, but deep melancholy can surface at any time during the course of the disease. Because the symptoms of depression mimic the symptoms of Alzheimer's, your loved one may require an evaluation for depression, which is explained more fully in chapter 13.

In addition to medications for Alzheimer's, there are medications for depression that can dramatically improve an individual's emotional state. Regular exercise and getting out into the sun and fresh air can help perk up a person with Alzheimer's who is also suffering from depression.

Talk therapy with a mental health expert combined with antidepressant medications is the most effective method for countering depression in the general population. But many professionals make the assumption that talk therapy cannot help in relieving depressive illness among those with advancing Alzheimer's who are unable to remember from session to session. However, my experience proved to me that it is worthwhile and can bring about relief. Some of the suggestions and tips in chapter 15 may prove helpful.

Now, here are two people, Frances and Connie, both plagued by anxiety and depression.

Meet Frances

Frances looked both fretful and frightened. Her face was drawn and had a quality that reminded me of a rubber band stretched too tight and about to snap. She darted from one person to another in her walker, the device that kept her from falling. She did stop to say hello, but before anyone could respond to her, she had quickly moved on.

The social worker had told me that when Frances first came to the unit, several of her friends had called to see how she was doing. But now no one called or visited her. Frances was being treated with an antidepressant and I thought that a support group might help her feel better.

After introducing myself with a smile, I asked, "Frances, how are you doing today?"

She looked at me with alarm in her small, gray eyes, and said, "I'm not sure."

"You seem to be edgy."

She mumbled something that made no sense to me. So I decided to ask, "Do you feel confused?"

"Yes."

"It must be nerve-racking to feel confused."

"It is." She acknowledged my comment in a low voice.

"How about joining our discussion group? We talk about things like what it's like to feel confused, and it might make you feel better."

"No, I don't think so. I have to wait here."

Week after week, I'd stop by and have the same conversation with her. One week, after she had declined to come into the group, I asked her anyway and added, "Frances, what do you have to lose? Try it out, and if you don't like it, you can leave." That worked.

She let me guide her to the room where the group met, still looking worried. I noticed her looking at the door once or twice, but she stayed.

She came to group for several weeks, always looking distracted. Once she settled in, however, she seemed interested in whatever was being discussed. But whenever I directed a question to her that related to the current theme, she'd respond by saying, "I don't know," or by speaking in mixed-up fragments of speech that were unrelated to the question.

I struggled to make some sense of what she'd said, but I rarely succeeded.

After several sessions, Frances began to smile occasionally and to look people in the eye. Her face became more expressive, and the worry lines on her forehead softened as she listened to what the others were saying. She appeared to be more relaxed.

The following week, the group meeting began with one member saying, "They told me my whole life that I am depressed. What is depression?

I replied, "That's a good question." I asked each person in the group, "What do you think depression is?

One individual said, "Depression is when you wake up feeling crabby and you don't know why."

"How do you deal with it?" I asked.

"I stay by myself, away from people, and pray that when I wake up the next day, I'll feel better."

Someone else commented, "Depression is when you cry and cry."

Then I turned to Frances and asked her if she ever felt depressed. To my utter surprise, she answered, with great conviction, "I think I have been more depressed in my life than I've ever admitted to myself."

Frances had spoken her first complete sentence to the group, a sentence filled with insight and self-appraisal.

. . . .

Lessons from Frances: Useful Tools and Related Comments

Frances's depression was also mixed with anxiety, which made it harder for me to reach her. However, never underestimate the power of persistence. That means don't give up on anyone. By visiting her regularly and always inviting her into the group, either I had become a familiar face to Frances or I'd worn her down. Although she never remembered me in the ordinary sense, she began to trust more and fear less. She'd finally agreed to attend only after I'd posed the question "What do you have to lose?" And I caught her on a good day. Some days were better for her than other days, just as it is for all of us.

When you see your loved one with Alzheimer's on a regular basis, you may become a person whom she can trust, even if she has forgotten your name or who you are. Respect her wishes if she doesn't want to talk at that moment. Try to engage her again a little later. Even if you don't succeed in getting a conversation going, she will perceive that you made the effort and sense that you care.

The fact that both of you may just sit together in silence counts. Read more about how to deal with quiet people who do not verbalize, despite your efforts, in chapter 13.

> **Tool 20: Be Persistent but Respectful**
>
> - It takes time for someone with Alzheimer's to sense that you are a friendly face.
>
> - Respect a no response, but ask again later.
>
> - Sharing silence is a way to connect.

Everyone who worked with Frances could see that she was anxious from the way she restlessly dashed from one person to another. She was probably afraid because she couldn't understand where she was or who she was. That would upset anyone. Putting myself into her shoes, I applied Tool 2, Show Empathy, realizing that she must be confused, and asking her if that was true. Frances acknowledged my comment, but she wasn't persuaded to attend the group until I gave her permission to leave if she didn't want to stay. Offering her a way out gave her a choice and provided reassurance.

Frances was included in every group discussion, regardless of whether her contribution made sense. Since no one knows exactly how much a person with Alzheimer's actually absorbs or thinks, treat her as if she does understand the gist of what you say.

> **Tool 21: Assume That Your Loved One Can Understand**
>
> - Assume that people are reachable, even if they seem uninterested or withdrawn. Don't give up. Keep using the tools.
>
> - Offer choices, issue invitations not demands, and support participation.
>
> - Your loved one may understand or remember more than you may think.

For the most part, group members were accepting of Frances and each other. As she began to feel safer with the group members, Frances appeared to become more comfortable, and so she became willing to attend the group regularly.

I was impressed that everyone had ideas about how to cope with depression. Evidently, depression was a familiar subject to everyone, even though it was rarely mentioned. If someone else in the group had not introduced the subject of depression, Frances may never have had the opportunity to gain insight into her life.

Introducing uncomfortable topics with your loved one may present her with the chance to talk about something that strikes a chord. On the other hand, you have to be ready to engage in such an exchange while not knowing how she may react.

As a psychologist, I urge you to bring up uncomfortable topics in the most general ways, because as you saw with Frances's example, it is preferable to talk about the issues that bother a person with advancing Alzheimer's rather than to just ignore them. For more information about depression, see chapter 13.

Tool 22: Check for Signs of Depression

- Observe whether your loved one is changing for the worse.

- Ask your loved one about feeling sad and be ready to discuss it.

- Have a professional assess your loved one for depression or illness.

When Francis made her insightful remark to the group about how depressed she had always been, it was the first time she had been as clear as a bell in her communication.

Meet Connie

Connie was a chocoholic. By using her good left arm to maneuver and keeping her left foot whizzing along, she knew how to make her wheelchair move rapidly. She did this when she wanted chocolate, hastening to the third-floor candy machines where she put a coin into the slot and received her reward: a chocolate candy bar. However, even chocolate provided her with only momentary relief from depression.

Her astute physician, noticing how she was always in motion, requested that I assess her.

"How are you doing, Connie?" I asked, after making the proper introductions.

"I don't know why I am in this place. I'm not crazy," she replied earnestly.

"This isn't a place for crazy people. It's a place to help people who have trouble getting around the way they used to," I explained.

"I can get along just fine. I can take care of myself," she retorted. Connie seemed oblivious to the paralysis of the right side of her body and other limitations that soon became apparent to me, which were the results of a stroke.

"How would you manage by yourself?" I countered, trying to see if, indeed, she could live on her own.

"I would just figure it out," she answered evasively, her eyes lowered.

"What would you need to do?"

"I don't know."

"Where would you live?"

"I don't know," she said again, her eyes not meeting mine.

"How would you feed yourself?"

"I don't know, but I would figure it out," she said, sounding annoyed.

When our talk came to the specifics of how she could take care of herself, Connie was stuck. Clearly, she didn't know how to take care of herself on her own. I could see that being in constant motion was her way of reacting to her intense anxiety and sadness about her plight. She was clueless about her deficits, where she was, and why she was here.

I told her, "It must be tough for you to be here when you feel you could manage on your own. Would you like someone to talk to you about this situation?" She agreed that would be okay with her, and she began individual therapy.

As the weeks went by, Connie's memory increasingly faltered. Her depression didn't get worse, but she had trouble completing a sentence, and that added to her frustration.

Several months after individual therapy ended, with her mood showing some improvement, I lost track of Connie. Then I discovered that she had been transferred to another ward because she could no longer move about on her own without losing her way. She also had forgotten how to use utensils to eat.

I visited her in the new ward where I saw a different Connie. In contrast to her previous anxious and unhappy demeanor, she smiled when I greeted her, even though it was apparent that she didn't recognize me. She sat as if glued to her wheelchair, no longer able to move herself independently but no longer restless. Hardly able to speak a word, Connie didn't say hello back to me, she only smiled. I asked her to join a group because I thought that some social stimulation might help her. She didn't answer but she didn't fight it.

I escorted her down the drab hallway. When we arrived, I offered her some hot chocolate, but she graciously said, "No, thank you." I gulped, realizing that she had lost her taste for chocolate, her favorite treat.

After several meetings, Connie began to respond with more than a smile, and she graduated to uttering fragmented phrases that I could piece together. She mentioned family members whom she had not spoken of at all when her memory was more intact. Connie took an interest in whatever topic was being discussed, and she always said something when I'd ask her to comment, even though it often was "I don't know." But she laughed when she said it. Her smile, laughter, and good humor cheered up the group.

For Connie, the advance of Alzheimer's had given her the ultimate relief from a depression that nothing else had been able to accomplish.

· ·

Lessons from Connie: Useful Tools and Related Comments

Connie never did understand why she was in this new, unfamiliar environment, and that alarmed her. She could only express dismay at her placement in a nursing home, which she saw as a place for "crazy" people. And she knew that she wasn't crazy. She had no idea that she had become unable to take care of herself. Any explanation I gave her did not convince her.

Some people with Alzheimer's don't realize that something is terribly amiss, that they have lost the skills they need to survive on their own. After all, the person with the illness is being asked to believe something about herself that contradicts her own perceptions, which was not only baffling for Connie, but depressing as well. She comforted herself with eating lots of chocolate.

It is very sad for someone to be in this position. If you confront her with the truth that she has deteriorated, she may become even more depressed by the reality. If you point out that she is receiving help, she looks at you as if you're crazy, declaring, "I don't need any help!" The only thing you can do is offer support by saying, "Yes. I know how hard this is for you. It's confusing and aggravating." Remember Tool 3, Use What You Know to Go with the Flow, and agree.

Tool 23: Avoid Confrontation

- Avoid confrontation. Do not argue.

- Be empathic with your loved one who may be unable to recognize his limitations.

- Acknowledge his reality by saying that, as hard as it is to believe, everyone is only trying to help. When he says that he doesn't need help, simply nod in agreement and say, "I know. I know."

In contrast to the first time I met Connie, when I saw her again she hardly spoke nor could she do anything for herself. However, Connie did begin to talk again when she was re-exposed to the ongoing stimulation of other people who addressed her as if she did understand. She was invited to give her input. You need to provide encouragement to your loved one, asking for her opinion even if she doesn't respond the first few times you try.

Your loved one may enter a phase of just sitting without uttering a word. He just cannot initiate and negotiate communicating. This is the time when it is incumbent on everyone to reach out and find the dots to connect. If we give up on someone at this stage, we have underestimated him and condemned him to a life of isolation. Again, see chapter 13 for additional discussion of what your loved one's persistent quiet may indicate.

Ironically, as her cognitive losses increased, Connie forgot that she had been depressed. Her memory loss gave her the relief from depression that neither chocolate nor treatment could provide.

CHAPTER 9

Who Are You Talking To?
Dealing with Delusions

Delusions or hallucinations appear in about half the cases of Alzheimer's as the disease progresses. Onset varies; some studies suggest that initially delusions materialize in 30 percent of the people with Alzheimer's, and the incidence increases as Alzheimer's advances (Fischer, Bozanovic-Sosic, and Norris 2004).

A *hallucination* is a false perception of something that an individual believes he actually sees, hears, or smells, and it is real to him, but it is not actually there. A *delusion* is a fixed belief held by someone even though there is no evidence that the belief is true. *Paranoia* is a type of delusion consisting of irrational suspiciousness and a belief that someone is going to harm him.

Paranoia is the most common type of delusion found in those with Alzheimer's. With advancing Alzheimer's, as confusion and memory loss increase, a person with the disease can become distrustful. Relatives or caregivers whom he no longer recognizes may be perceived as strangers who may hurt him. After all, how can someone who sees an "unfamiliar" person in his environment not be suspicious? Furthermore, the help the caregiver provides with bathing or dressing can be seen as an unwelcome intrusion. It is hard to understand that your loved one may mistrust you, but that may be the case.

Treatment is complicated for a person with Alzheimer's who has developed psychotic symptoms. If the person poses no risk to himself or others, current trends lean toward not medicating to treat the symptoms. Instead, behavioral interventions may work; see chapter 15 for details. In the more difficult situations when a person may threaten to harm himself or others, antipsychotic medication can be prescribed, but it is recommended as a last resort, because any medication may have side effects. If you have concerns in this regard, ask a physician who specializes in geriatric psychiatry if your loved one is a candidate for medication.

New areas of exploration are emerging from reports that when a person is remembering a scenario, she is reliving the incident in her brain (Carey 2008a). Perhaps that contributes to why false beliefs are so convincing for the person who holds them: she is utterly certain that what she believes is indisputably true, as you will see with Sylvia.

Meet Sylvia

I saw a hunched over, chubby woman sitting in a chair with a beatific half smile on her face, her eyes glazed over, staring out into space. I knew that she suffered from a recurring delusion that her mother was alive and well. She was often heard muttering to herself, saying, "Mom, that's a good idea."

"Sylvia, may I interrupt you?" I said gently. I reintroduced myself and sat catty-corner on the edge of her bed, hoping I could get her attention without startling her. She widened her eyes, blinked, raised her eyebrows, and smiled, but didn't say anything. I asked, "How about joining our discussion group?" By that time, she had been a regular attendee.

After hesitating, she softly replied, "Oh, all right. Where should I go?"

"Don't worry. I'll take you. It's right down the hall."

Sylvia could no longer initiate any actions without hands-on supervision. She was happy to be guided and was always agreeable with staff, unless she was engaged in a heated discussion with her mother.

I helped Sylvia stand up and offered her my arm. It was a long walk down the hallway to the meeting room, and although she had looked solid, I noticed that her arthritic hands and fingers were gnarled and shaking when she took my arm, and that she placed one foot in front of the other unsteadily.

How can someone appear to be hearty and frail at the same time? I wondered.

She inched along, leaning heavily on me. I found myself walking so slowly that I had to watch my step. After what seemed an interminably long time, we entered the room and I led her to an armchair. She let go of my hand and, wobbly, sat down with a thud. Whew! I thought.

Although she'd agreed to use an audio amplifier, it was hard for Sylvia to stay awake in the group. I had to rouse her out of her reverie before I could ask her a question. Whenever I did, she would answer, "I don't know."

Occasionally, under her breath, Sylvia muttered a comment about what someone else had said. I would ask her to repeat her remark, but either she couldn't or wouldn't. From the little that I could hear, her reactions were right in line with the topic we were discussing.

Whenever we spoke about mothers, Sylvia would sit up straighter. When I asked her whether she missed her mother, Sylvia would look at me incredulously and say, "But Mother is here with me now." And she would turn her head, whispering something to her mother.

I said, "So she is."

. . . .

Lessons from Sylvia: Useful Tools and Related Comments

I approached Sylvia cautiously, not wanting to startle her. She responded.

Sylvia was convinced that her mother was alive and with her. It appeared to give her great comfort to have her mother at her side, even if they did have a spat once in a while. I thought about Tool 4, Agree. Interestingly, her delusion became a vehicle for interacting with others, and she nodded yes or no when they spoke about their mothers. The "advice" her mother gave her in the moment may have been Sylvia's recollections of what her mother used to tell her; the delusion served as a reminder.

Sylvia's attitude showed me that even a false belief can serve as a connection when you pause to explore it. Delusions notwithstanding, those with Alzheimer's can still make comments appropriate to the present moment.

Tool 24: Use the Delusion

- Interact with your loved one about the delusional material she expresses.

- See the delusion as an expression of thoughts and wishes.

- Explore a delusion as you would any fragments you hear.

- Accept the delusion as part of her reality.

I saw no reason to challenge Sylvia's perception of her mother's presence. It gave her comfort.

CHAPTER 10

How Do I Look?
Appearance Still Counts

Most people go to great lengths to project an attractive appearance. The way a person looks shapes the way she sees herself and can make her feel better when she is happy with the result. How a person presents herself to the outside world is part of her self-image. Her appearance, along with her deeds, affects how she sees herself and contributes to her self-esteem, a critical component of psychological well-being. Researchers point out that self-esteem increases when an individual feels appreciated, accepted, and respected (Gerritsen et al. 2007). As an extension of our identity, our appearance can improve the way we feel about ourselves despite inner turmoil.

An individual with Alzheimer's may be very much aware of his appearance if it was important to him in the past. Note that men can be just as concerned about how they look as women are. The stories about Jane and Mario below demonstrate, among other things, that appearances count.

Meet Jane

When she first attended the group, I did a double take: there before me sat a diminutive reincarnation of my late mother-in-law. How could two people look so much alike, one a miniature of the other? They even shared a penchant for scarves to cover their similar gray, wavy hair. The shape of their faces and their expressions were identical. Jane even spoke with the same pauses and phraseology. However, this elderly woman was cheerful, whereas my mother-in-law had rarely cracked a smile. And Jane weighed about 100 pounds, but my late mother-in-law had weighed in at about 250.

Jane's eyes sparkled with merriment. She seemed very cheerful for someone with hallucinations and delusions that may have predated Alzheimer's. She had managed to build a small but solid life in the community. In the group, Jane was a live wire, chuckling as she repeated confabulated stories of her life, stories that even the others sensed were confusing. However, everyone appreciated her disjointed but lively tales in spite of the confusion. I would tell her, "Jane, you have a wonderful outlook that delights us all!" When I told her that, she would smile appreciatively.

Every group session began with me asking each person to state her name, since announcing one's name proclaims one's identity. Jane would reply with a smile, "I'm just plain Jane!" Of course, other group members would chime in and say, "You're not plain!" when I'd ask them if they agreed.

One day we had a visitor who had blonde hair. I asked the usual question: "How are you doing today?"

When it was Jane's turn, she answered by saying, wistfully, "I miss being a blonde. Now I am gray. I just loved being blonde. I never wore a head scarf then. I wish I could be a blonde again!"

Not only was that news to all of us, but we were surprised that Jane was so coherent. Her comments set off a lively discussion about one's appearance. I had not realized that it was still so important to these women. They sounded like a bunch of ladies chatting during lunch at a restaurant. From the way Jane spoke, it seemed true that, at least for her, blondes do have more fun.

Amid the laughter, someone quietly said, "I want my appearance to be a good person on the inside." A hush fell as each person assimilated that piece of wisdom.

. . . .

Lessons from Jane: Useful Tools and Related Comments

From Jane, I learned that we can assume that people with Alzheimer's and other psychotic mannerisms can still care about their appearance. My first reaction to Jane was based on how she looked. Don't be surprised if your loved one with Alzheimer's reminds you of someone you knew or perhaps how that person was at an earlier time. You can tell your loved one that she reminds you of someone else, or you can process it later with someone you trust. I chose not to speak of it and kept the focus on Jane. She had a vibrant personality and a sense of humor that appealed to all of us. However, on some level everyone in the group seemed aware that something else besides forgetfulness was amiss with Jane, and yet they accepted her idiosyncrasies.

Group members disputed Jane's description of herself as "plain," and they seemed to recognize it had been a self-deprecating remark. Their responses demonstrated how supportive they were. When they offered positive feedback to Jane, she beamed and felt appreciated.

The blonde-haired visitor caught Jane's eye and reminded her of her wish for her own blonde hair color, an issue that evidently meant a lot to her. The external stimulus, a new face, resulted in a connection. Jane expressed herself in a sensible manner, a rare occurrence. I had no idea that Jane (and nearly everyone else) had such strong opinions about how they looked.

The way you appear might have an impact on your loved one as well, awakening her own ideas about her own attire, hair style, makeup, or accessories. What a fun connection to explore. Be sensitive to her wishes and supportive of her ideas; it will enhance her self-esteem and make you both feel better.

Tool 25: Self-Image Counts

- Realize that her appearance may still be important to her.

- Involve your loved one in choosing what to wear.

- Offer an either-or choice, to simplify decision making.

- Compliment her to support her selection. Enjoy the experience.

The final comment indicated that "the way one is on the inside is what's really important." Pockets of wisdom can be sprinkled throughout your loved one's brain despite advancing Alzheimer's.

Meet Mario

Mario was an elegant gentleman who had retired from a prominent position in the diplomatic corps. Every day he wore a sports jacket and a fedora perched rakishly on his head. Mario would tip his hat whenever he greeted the ladies, even though he was wheelchair-bound and had advancing Alzheimer's. Mario liked to flirt.

His wife visited him faithfully twice a week and he remembered her. Mario even knew her name. He was always asking for her. She spoke to him in Italian, his native tongue, and she brought him his favorite foods.

When I asked him to join the group, he'd reply in Italian.

"Use English, Signore, use English!" I said, not understanding another word of Italian.

"I cannot come," he'd answer in English.

"Why not?"

"I am waiting for my wife," he would explain, not realizing that she had visited him earlier in the day.

"I'll see to it that your wife will find us when she comes. We'll be just down the hall." Mario would hesitate and then agree, his face looking a little doubtful.

I included Mario in all the discussions, and when it was his turn to comment, he would say something completely unrelated. At other times, he would simply say, "Sure. Of course," sounding congenial but looking as though he hadn't grasped the gist of what anyone had said. I never heard him make any relevant remarks, but he often had a smile on his face.

I wondered whether he would have an easier time communicating in Italian. However, when I checked this out with a staff member who spoke Italian, I found out that he wasn't comprehensible in that language either.

When the subject of careers came up in group, Mario did not participate directly until I said, "Mario, you have met many important people in your life."

"Ah, yes. Ah, yes," was his response.

One day I approached him to introduce myself yet again, and he looked up at me from under the brim of his hat. Slowly, a look of recognition lit up his face and he exclaimed, with wonder, "I know you! I know you!" his face joyful as he gave a jaunty tug on the brim of his fedora.

It made my day.

. . . .

Lessons from Mario: Useful Tools and Related Comments

Mario had been required to dress appropriately all those years he'd worked in diplomacy. He knew how to interact socially with all types of people. Mario valued looking well dressed, and his wife informed the staff of his preferences. Respecting his wishes contributed to his self-esteem, as suggested in Tool 25, Self-Image Counts.

Mario could still charm the people he met, especially the women. His well-developed social skills helped him relate to others. He responded to anyone who greeted him with a smile and a tug on his fedora.

Tool 26: Capitalize on Remaining Social Skills

- Basic social amenities such as "Hello, how are you?" and "Thank you" are bridges for either of you to connect.

- Keep on interacting even if he doesn't make much sense.

Mario didn't remember much, but he knew his wife. The fact that he did remember her was a great source of comfort for them both. He was confused about the time of day and couldn't remember that his wife had visited him earlier. When I approached him, I respected Mario's concern about possibly missing his wife's visit, and I acknowledged his reality, an application of Tool 3, Use What You Know to Go with the Flow. He wasn't quite convinced someone would tell his wife where he was, but he came to the group anyway, after hearing from me the reassurance that he would be summoned when his wife arrived.

Tool 27: Be Reassuring

- It is important to acknowledge, respect, and address his concerns, whatever the situation.

- Reassurance can reduce anxiety and induce cooperation.

I thought that Mario might be at a disadvantage in that those around him didn't speak Italian. One's native language is retained in one's long-term memory. Frequently, a person will revert to the language of his youth because he forgets his second language, which he learned later. I was lucky that Mario could still speak English.

I checked to see if Mario might be less confused if he was addressed in Italian and discovered that it really didn't matter which language was spoken. Mario made unintelligible comments in Italian, as well as in English. Using English to speak to me was a sign that he remembered I did not speak Italian, and wanted to connect.

Tool 28: Consider Your Loved One's Native Language

- Your loved one may remember and understand communication in his native language rather than English.

- Your loved one may have difficulty understanding English that is spoken with an accent.

The one person Mario was clear about identifying was his wife. Your loved one may have trouble remembering the names of the people he loves. It took a long time, but when Mario finally recognized me, although not by name, I was delighted.

Tool 29: Be Prepared for Nonrecognition

- Be prepared for your loved one to forget your name or who you are.

- Understand that this loss of memory is beyond his control.

- He may still remember someone important to him.

Use the tools and your loved one may finally remember that you are someone special. Unfortunately, as Alzheimer's progresses, the ability to recognize a wife, daughter, son, relative, or friend gradually disappears. It is heartbreaking when that happens. Furthermore, because your loved one with Alzheimer's may feel afraid because he is among "strangers," he may react with suspicion. In some way, he knows that something is amiss and that he has upset you, but he doesn't know why.

When a loved one can no longer recognize you, you can receive some consolation in knowing that he might intuit that you are someone special in his life, even though he cannot identify you per se. Often relatives and friends become so discouraged when they are not recognized that they gradually stop conversing with the person as Alzheimer's advances. Gather up the courage to keep on trying. When you read chapter 14, you will see that there is some good news about memory and Alzheimer's.

CHAPTER 11

But Where Do I Go? Memory Inconsistencies

As brain cells disintegrate, pieces of memories stored in various areas of the brain may survive, especially those from long ago. In Alzheimer's, intermittent memory lapses gradually become frequent; the person may go from not being able to remember minutes, hours, and weeks before the present moment to forgetting what happened months or years ago. In terms of expressing himself, your loved one may appear to remember one moment, and in the next moment he may draw a blank. No wonder it's confusing for you both. Chapters 14 and 15 explain more about memory issues and Alzheimer's.

Edith's memory fluctuated, as you will see in the following account.

Meet Edith

"Edith will be a challenge," I thought to myself. Although I approached her in a friendly manner, I expected that Edith, who had been described to me as occasionally irascible and suspicious, would be difficult to engage. When I entered her room, she was busy poring over the daily newspaper.

"Excuse me, do you mind if I say hello?"

Edith looked up and said, "Of course."

After introducing myself, I said, "So, what's new in the world?" pointing at the newspaper.

"I don't know. But I enjoy reading the newspaper over and over again, because I cannot remember what I've just read." she replied, conversationally.

"Keep on reading, if you like, and enjoy."

"I can always read it again later."

To my surprise, I found that Edith was charming, although week after week she refused to attend the group. I continued to visit her anyway. We would chat. Then one week she said that she would come. She stood up, using her walker, and followed me into the group room. I thought that either the medication she was taking to counteract her suspiciousness was working or perhaps she had started to trust me.

I focused on her during her first session, asking her to introduce herself and to say something about her background. To my surprise, she provided a lengthy answer: "I fled from my family and my country in Europe in the late 1930s at the age of seventeen."

I asked why and she answered, "I never really got along with my mother and decided I should strike out on my own. I went to England and learned English as I became a nurse.

After remaining in England throughout the war, I came to America, where I continued to work until I retired."

What an unexpected recitation, I thought, amazed that she was so open and able to tell such a complete story, one that she had never mentioned before. Unsuccessful in my attempt to have her say more about what not getting along with her mother meant, I commented, "What a courageous path you took, Edith. Why did you become a nurse?"

"Because of the war, you see, and England needed nurses," she said, matter-of-factly.

"Would you have studied nursing anyway?"

"No. I always wanted to be a doctor. But you see there was no time for that because of the war, and nurses were needed."

With that, Edith asked me about my training and was impressed that I had a Ph.D.

"So you are a doctor," she said, with admiration mixed in with a little envy.

At times, Edith could be bitingly critical of group members. "You don't know what you are talking about," she said one day when someone had expressed an opinion different from her own.

"Ouch, that hurt," I said, trying to ease the impact of her insensitivity. "Some people have different opinions." I hoped to take the sting out of her remarks.

She retorted, "But it's true!"

I replied, "A wise person once told me that honesty without compassion can be a form of cruelty." She remained silent until the next time someone stated an opinion that differed from her own.

As time went by, although she still had an occasional flare-up, Edith became more amiable. Whenever I provided a snack during our session, she would say to me, "You should have someone helping you. You are a doctor, and you shouldn't have to serve us ice cream. Can I help you?"

Surprised that she remembered my title but not knowing how she could be of help, I answered, "Thanks, Edith, but I can manage."

She continued to come to the group and began to linger as I helped others to leave the room at the end of the session. One day, when I came back for someone else, I found her standing in her walker and moving around the room, collecting all the empty ice cream cups and placing them in the trash can.

"I see I have someone to help me after all," I said, appreciatively. She smiled with satisfaction, happy that she had figured out a way to assist me. When all the soiled cups were dropped into the trash can, she turned to me and said, "Now, how do I get to my room?"

. . . .

Lessons from Edith: Useful Tools and Related Comments

Edith was in the middle stages of Alzheimer's disease. See chapter 13 for more information about how the phases of Alzheimer's unfold.

Before my first meeting with Edith, I applied Tool 3, Use What You Know to Go with the Flow, and learned about her background. Discovering that she could be paranoid helped me to approach her in a way that was totally nonthreatening. With persistency and respect, and the application of Tool 20, Be Persistent but Respectful, we finally connected. She began to trust me.

Edith could still process complex thoughts about her past, and she was able to recall noteworthy events that had left an indelible imprint on her mind. She put together a narrative in proper sequence, outlining decisions she had made sixty years earlier. She remembered and understood more than I would have thought possible, exemplifying the rationale behind Tool 21, Assume That Your Loved One Can Understand. She was proud of the gumption she had shown when she left her family at such a young age to carve out a life for herself. And she regretted that she had never become a physician. Her story reflected how intact she was, in one dimension.

Your loved one may recall a specific time or situation with great clarity.

Tool 30: Expect That Some Things Are Remembered

- Your loved one may remember an event that has a strong emotional association.

- A coherent retelling occasionally may arise.

Edith could be intolerant and insensitive to other's people's ideas and feelings. By using Tool 7, Don't Take an Unkind Remark Too Seriously, I was able to act as a buffer to soften the impact of her harsh remarks, sensing that she may have been capable of understanding on some level.

Edith was sensitive to social class distinctions and to the nuances of the doctor-nurse relationship. I was surprised when she stated that it was not appropriate for me to serve ice cream. Edith let me know that she had a desire to be useful. Not only did she remember that I was a doctor, but she wanted to help me, which was a reenactment of her role as a nurse.

We may mistakenly assume that the limitations of a loved one render her incapable of contributing in any way. Yet contributing gives a person a sense of purpose and enhances self-esteem. Involve your loved one in activities to make her feel important, especially by participating in basic routines. Edith took the lead. She taught me a valuable lesson.

Tool 31: Learn from Your Loved One

- Listen and learn.

- Find ways to help your loved one feel useful.

For Edith to become bewildered about how to go her room was doubly significant since her room was right next door. That's how inconsistent memory can be for someone with Alzheimer's, but the moments she can remember are precious.

CHAPTER 12

How Do I Say Good-Bye? Leaving Until the Next Time

One of the hardest things to do is to say good-bye to a loved one after spending time together. If you care for a loved one at home, this may be difficult as well. He might not want you to leave, even though you have arranged for someone else to be with him. Ideally, the person who will help you may be familiar to him, but you may have a different caregiver or a relative or friend whom he does not remember. Let them both know that you have to leave, but that you'll be back in a specified time. Reassure your loved one that you will return, and acknowledge your understanding of his reaction. Use Tool 2, Show Empathy, listen, and be kind.

If he reacts positively, make your exit. If he is apprehensive, involve the three of you in a favorite activity. You could listen to music, do an art project, or discuss meaningful photographs, and be sure to have the other caregiver participate. When you see that your loved one is involved, say, "See you later," and depart.

Whether your loved one is at home or in a nursing facility, first give a ten-minute and then a five-minute warning that you will soon go away. This will allow time for your loved one to express her feelings about you leaving. Talking about upset feelings is a healthy way to cope.

The following story about Madeline highlights the issues that may arise when saying good-bye.

Meet Madeline

I watched her waddling down the hallway in front of me, her flaming orange-and-blue flowered muumuu sliding across a large rear end, back and forth, as she lumbered along toward the group room. Clop–drag, clop–drag. The sound of her walker hitting the floor echoed the extraordinary effort she made. But she was walking.

After what seemed to be an unbearable amount of time, she maneuvered herself into the room and reached her destination: a large leather chair with two wooden arms. I wondered if she'd be able to figure out how to execute the complexities of seating herself without falling. She had Alzheimer's plus worn-out, arthritic knees. The simple act of sitting down, something we all do without any thought, was a major challenge.

I watched her apprehensively, resisting the urge to help her. I knew that the unit's staff would not have permitted her to use a walker unless she had demonstrated that she actually could, but I was still worried.

Madeline came to a stop in front of the chair. I held my breath. Slowly, her right hand let go of the walker's side railing. She bent forward, all 300 pounds of her, and reached for the arm of the chair. Then she removed her left hand from the walker railing and grabbed the other arm of the chair. So far, so good. Madeline was on her own.

She moved her right hand to the back of the chair and heaved herself around, her rear end directly over the seat of the chair. Plop! She made it! I let out my breath slowly. She suddenly looked up and saw me staring. Her face broke into a triumphant smile, in contrast to its customary vacant look, and her eyes glistened with pride.

After the others arrived, Madeline's face resumed its usual blank stare. I had wondered whether she would connect to me and to the others. But whenever I addressed her or asked for an opinion, the mask lifted and she became animated, making sense.

Six weeks before I retired from my job, I announced to the group that I was leaving, telling them the news in advance, as I would for any therapy group, even if it seemed that no one remembered what we discussed from week to week. I was hoping that they could start to process my impending departure, as it is important from a psychological standpoint to give every member of a group plenty of time to say good-bye to someone whom she will not see again.

Madeline looked grief-stricken. She said, "You can't do that."

Despite my training, I squirmed. I had prepared myself for negative reactions, but I had not expected that one. Finally, I said, "I know. It's a shock. I am retiring." No one else made any comment.

After the session, I informed the unit's staff members that I had told the group about my leaving, and that they might notice an increase in depression or anxiety within the members of the group, particularly Madeline. They looked at me skeptically.

Later that week, when I checked back, the nurse in charge told me that, indeed, Madeline did look depressed; she was staring off into space more than usual.

Five weeks before my departure, I brought up my retirement date to the group again (as I would do for the remaining weeks). This time, there was more discussion. In response to my question about how members felt about me leaving, Madeline said, "You are always smiling. Just seeing you makes us feel good."

I told them that they made me feel good, as well. I meant it.

When I wondered aloud if they were angry with me for going away, inviting their reactions because anger is a normal response to a leader who leaves, they looked incredulous. They made comments such as "But you are never angry with us" and "I don't think you get angry at anyone."

I felt self-conscious.

As the weeks went by, I continued to raise the topic of my retirement at every session. At the next to last session, Madeline commented, "What I love about you is that you are always the same and always stay the same." "I love all of you too," I replied, realizing that I did.

At the last session, I announced that someone else would try to continue leading the group once a month. Madeline shook her head from side to side and said, "But you are irreplaceable. You are one of us. You treat us as if you are one of us. You talk to us and never talk down to us."

Surprised and touched, I couldn't think of a good response to that, but my facial expression was more telling than anything I could have said. Finally, I said, "That is so touching. It's hard for me to say good-bye, too. I will miss all of you."

As the close of that final session drew near, I went around the room and gave each person a hug, after first checking that it was all right to do so, reassuring each one that I would never forget how special she was. And now you know how special they are, too.

. . . .

Lessons from Madeline: Useful Tools and Related Comments

When we see someone executing a task unsteadily, it's hard to know what that person can still do. I had been worried about Madeline's stability, even though she was using a walker. My instinct told me to interfere and help her, especially when I could help her down the hallway in half the time. The uncertainty of not knowing if she could walk using the walker filled me with anxiety, especially for her safety. It's a difficult call, but I realized that to deprive someone of doing what she is still capable of doing is to rob her of her dignity. I had to fight my own anxious feelings to allow Madeline to get to the room under her own steam. Afterward, I was glad that I did.

If I had butted in, I would have been dealing with my own nervousness under the guise of helping her, undermining her confidence and the collective wisdom of the unit staff members who had okayed her walking. You too may be facing decisions about whether or not to interfere with a task your loved one can barely do. Seek assistance from an occupational or physical therapist who can observe your loved one and determine what is safe for him to continue to do.

> **Tool 32: Let Her Do What She Still Can Do**
>
> • After consulting with an expert, permit your loved one to do what she is still capable of doing, even if it's nerve-racking for you to watch.
>
> • Oversee the task.
>
> • Give her time to accomplish the task. Be patient.
>
> • Be aware of your own feelings and think before you act.

You don't have to leave abruptly; give some lead-in time before you depart. I allowed six weeks for the process of saying good-bye; you can devote ten minutes to remind your loved one that you'll soon be on your way but will return. Fortunately, you, in contrast to me, will come again. I couldn't. I had to tell them I would not return.

It's okay for your loved one to say that she doesn't want you to go. Apply Tool 2, Show Empathy. Let her know that you know how she feels, and that you feel that way, too. I resisted the urge to say, "Oh, you'll be all right. Other people are still here to take care of you," because that would have put dealing with my own discomfort ahead of acknowledging her feelings. However, you still need an outlet to express yourself. Talk about it with someone else.

> **Tool 33: Do Not Underestimate Feelings About Saying Good-Bye**
>
> - She has feelings about you leaving, and so do you.
>
> - Let her know that you will be leaving. First tell her ten minutes before leaving, and then five minutes before you go.
>
> - She recognizes and appreciates kindness.
>
> - Accept her feelings.

I learned a lot about how much heart and thinking ability Madeline and all the group members had left, even with their profound memory loss. Once again, they showed me they were much more aware than I had thought they would be. I realized that above all else, it's important to treat your loved one with Alzheimer's as an equal.

We all had connected and communicated, and we knew it. Love permeated the atmosphere whenever we met. Now you have the same opportunity. Use the tools to establish a connection with your loved one, who will connect right back with you. Your relationship lives on.

PART II

Delving Deeper

CHAPTER 13

Back to Basics: About
Alzheimer's and Dementia

You are not alone. Currently in the United States, approximately 10 million unpaid caregivers shoulder the burden of care for loved ones: the 5.2 million people with Alzheimer's. The number of cases of Alzheimer's in the United States may triple by midcentury (Alzheimer's Association 2009). At this time, there are more than 24 million people with Alzheimer's worldwide (Kanter 2008).

What exactly is Alzheimer's? The average person has a great deal of confusion and misunderstanding about the disease, so if someone you know has Alzheimer's, you really need to know the facts: Alzheimer's disease is the most prevalent form of dementia. It afflicts people from all walks of life, from professors to migrant farmworkers.

There is no clear-cut understanding about why some people develop Alzheimer's and others do not. The greatest risk factor is age: the older you are, the greater the probability of onset. Less than 5 percent of cases occur in people under the age of sixty-five (Alzheimer's Association 2009).

Alzheimer's strikes both men and women, but because women live longer than men, as women age the number of women with Alzheimer's increases: 55 to 60 percent of all cases are women; 40 to 45 percent are men (Cummings and Cole 2002). Countries with lower life expectancies have a lower incidence of the disease.

There is no one simple cause (Rikkert, Teunisse, and Vernooij-Dassen 2005). Over the years, studies have suggested that Alzheimer's is caused by a combination of factors that can bring about the onset of the disease. Research has shown that there is a genetic component in some cases, especially in the early-onset population, but no one can point to one specific answer at this time (Alzheimer's Association 2009). To further complicate matters, another type of dementia that may require additional treatment often coexists with Alzheimer's. Conditions such as delirium, depression, or even another illness could be the culprit, alone or in addition to Alzheimer's.

However, before we can sort these out, it is important to take a closer look at the relationship between dementia and Alzheimer's disease.

Dementia

Dementia is a deterioration of memory, intellect, judgment, and emotional functioning. According to some neuroscientists (Glick and Dudson 2005), memory deficits fall into the following subcategories:

1. **Immediate:** Unable to recall an event one to two seconds later.

2. **Short-term:** Unable to recall an event after several seconds but less than a minute.

3. **Recent:** Unable to recall events that occurred minutes, days, weeks, or months previously.

4. **Long-term:** Unable to recall events or information from several minutes ago to hours, days, months, or years before.

5. **Remote:** Unable to recall events from decades earlier, although *episodic remote memory*, which is associated with strong emotional reactions tied to a specific situation, may be retained longer.

The assessment of memory loss requires the expertise of a neuropsychologist or *geropsychiatrist* (a psychiatrist who specializes in the care of older people), who can distinguish between these overlapping groups.

The loss of immediate to long-term memory is a frightening and perplexing experience for the person who cannot remember as well as for that person's relatives and caregivers. The person with dementia:

- displays confusion and memory loss, especially for short-term and recent events

- has difficulty following a conversation, finding the right words to say, and answering questions appropriately

- is unaware of safety issues and may not be able to figure out how to navigate to a familiar place without getting lost

- has difficulty learning new information or skills

When an individual develops dementia, it is a signal that brain cells, the overseers of all aspects of the human body and mind, have become damaged in several possible ways. Oxygen deprivation, an interruption of blood flow, direct injury, or an unnatural breakdown of protein can cause the brain to malfunction and can interfere with communication within the brain, breaking the circuitry. The change in abilities and behavior of the person with dementia can be sudden or gradual and can create frustration and anxiety for family members, as well as for the loved individual.

What Distinguishes Dementia from Sporadic Forgetting

If Joe forgets a telephone number he knew before, that is a common experience that falls into the category of occasional forgetfulness. However, if Joe not only forgets the number but also forgets how to use a telephone, that is unusual, and dementia may be the cause.

Based on the official guidelines for the diagnosis of dementia (American Psychiatric Association 1994), the phrase "one plus one" is a language shortcut you can use to recognize the onset of dementia. The first "one" represents memory loss, which is characteristic of most types of dementia. The forgetfulness usually starts with an inability to recall something that occurred recently. Using Joe and the telephone as an example, the second "one" could be one or more of the following:

- Having difficulty with the ability to plan, organize, or figure out what to do, such as Joe not knowing how to use a telephone. This is called a disturbance in *executive functioning*.

- Knowing it is a telephone, but not being able to pick up the receiver to carry out the complex muscular movements, even with the physical capability of doing so. This is an example of *apraxia*.

- Seeing the phone clearly as an object but not being able to recognize it is a telephone, perhaps misidentifying it as an unrelated object, or using another object such as a flashlight as if it were a telephone. Oliver Sacks (1987) describes this condition, called *agnosia*, in *The Man Who Mistook His Wife for a Hat*.

- Seeing the telephone but being unable to process the information in the speech center of the brain, resulting in an inability to say the word or substituting another word, such as "bone" for "phone." This language disturbance is called *aphasia*.

Mild Cognitive Impairment

People usually first seek help for troubling memory loss. If intermittent memory loss is the only feature present, a specialist might diagnose *mild cognitive impairment*, a condition that may lead to Alzheimer's disease (Petersen 2007, 2008). All told, almost one-half of those with mild cognitive impairment will develop Alzheimer's within the first five years after diagnosis.

Types of Dementia

Alzheimer's disease accounts for 70 percent of all cases of dementia (Alzheimer's Association 2009). Before going into detail about Alzheimer's itself, it is important to know about the other kinds of dementia, which can exist alone or in combination with Alzheimer's.

- *Vascular dementia,* also called *multi-infarct dementia,* accounts for 20 percent of all dementias. In contrast to Alzheimer's, which has a gradual onset, vascular dementia usually produces a sudden change in memory ability. *Circulatory* or *blood vessel disease* can cause an interruption in the flow of blood in the brain, precipitating strokes or the death of brain cells due to a lack of oxygen. After each occurrence of additional blood flow blockage or bleeding in the brain, the dementia may get worse. Other neurological symptoms and physiological impairments may accompany the cognitive problems.

- *Lewy body dementia* is similar to Alzheimer's, but usually starts at a younger age with symptoms such as shakiness, unsteadiness, delusions, and hallucinations. Lewy bodies are abnormal clusters of protein that accumulate in many areas of the brain.

- *Substance-induced dementia* may develop after years of excessive alcohol consumption, recreational or long-term use of drugs, or exposure to toxic substances. Occasionally, it is partially reversible after abstinence from the causative agent.

- Dementia may accompany other medical or neurological conditions such as a head injury or a blow to the brain, cardiac insufficiency or cardiac arrest, or breathing difficulties. Damage may result due to destroyed brain cells or to the reduced flow of oxygen to the brain.

- *Frontotemporal dementia* involves cell damage in the front and sides of the brain. Memory problems may not surface at the beginning. Instead, personality changes, apathy, disinhibition, compulsive behaviors, and a lack of empathy appear, with consistent memory loss not evident until later in the course of the disease.

- *Mixed dementia* is any combination of the types listed above. And that makes accurate diagnosis more challenging.

In addition to the classification criteria, it is important for professionals who make the diagnosis and for those of us who interact daily with patients to remember that dementia happens to a person, a self. We should always keep in mind that the unique self brings its own history, which has an impact on how people deal with the news of the diagnosis (Clare 2003). Alzheimer's is about a person, not just a disease.

The Role of Delirium and Depression in Dementia

Memory loss and mental confusion can also be a sign of delirium or depression, since many physical and psychological disorders start with confusion, memory loss, or acting "crazy." One of the distinguishing signs is how rapidly the symptoms appear.

Problems with memory that suddenly surface in minutes or over the course of a day or two may signal the onset of a stroke but could also indicate *delirium*, a brief and temporary loss of awareness of reality due to illness, infection, surgery, medication, sleep loss, dehydration, or malnutrition. People with delirium are confused, may become incoherent, and sometimes see things that are not really there, as in a visual hallucination. The symptoms of delirium usually reverse when the underlying medical problems are managed successfully.

The typical symptoms of depression are sadness, withdrawal, agitation, restlessness, irritability, angry outbursts, interrupted eating or sleeping patterns, and loss of energy for or interest in everyday affairs. However, confusion and forgetfulness may also be present, which can make the depression look like dementia when actually it is a pseudodementia brought on by the depression. After treatment for depression, memory and awareness return to normal. On the other hand, when someone with dementia becomes depressed, his usual befuddled state abruptly worsens. After managing the depression, some of the symptoms subside, but the underlying dementia remains.

Alzheimer's Disease

Alzheimer's disease is a progressive, degenerative, and irreversible brain disorder that eventually affects almost every aspect of the individual's mind, personality, health, lifestyle, and relationships. The person just isn't herself.

The Brain's Role

The brain is made up of billions of tiny cells, called *neurons*, each with an extension, or axon, that releases small amounts of chemicals through tiny fingerlike projections called *dendrites*, which fire an electron, sending a message to the dendrites of the next cell. The cell-to-cell communication creates the foundation for thinking and remembering. With Alzheimer's, a huge number of the brain cells break down into fragments of protein that form clusters, called *plaques*.

In addition, the protein in the long extensions of the axon breaks into pieces that interweave into structures called *tangles*. These tangles interrupt the flow of the information in the transport network from one cell to the next (Kanter 2008). The brain begins to shrink. The symptoms of Alzheimer's unfold.

When Alzheimer's is present, there is a gradual but obvious deterioration in doing one's job or talking with people appropriately and effortlessly. The person afflicted may be in the middle of doing something, and then not remember what she has to do next, and is unable to complete what she started. She cannot recall events that happened months, days, hours, or even two or three minutes before, even though she may remember information from a long time ago.

This translates into problems with day-to-day living, from paying bills to brushing teeth. The person with Alzheimer's may forget what day it is, or even where he is. He may not remember things we all take for granted and may also have trouble learning anything new. Confusion, fatigue, and embarrassment over his declining memory create a loss of interest in the activities he used to enjoy. Emotionally, stressful situations may trigger uncharacteristic outbursts of anger. Gradually, over months and years, memory problems and mental confusion escalate. Gait, balance, or coordination problems eventually develop.

Personality

Alzheimer's is stressful for everyone involved. Personality may change. From boorish to gentle, sweet to angry, the disposition of a person with Alzheimer's may shift away from its lifetime pattern or vacillate from one extreme to the other. Relaxed people can become anxious; stubborn people can become docile. Even when the personality stays the same, the person may still seem somehow different. Often someone with Alzheimer's is unaware of the extent of his deficits and lacks insight into his condition.

Within the range of normal relationships, the individual may have always been the predictable parent, spouse, grandparent, sibling, relative, or friend. Who could imagine the profound changes that take place with Alzheimer's and how they affect relatives and friends, and the person with the disease himself?

What It Is Like to Have Alzheimer's

Here is a picture of what life may be like for someone with advancing Alzheimer's:

Imagine waking up in the morning and not knowing where you are or who you are. You feel confused. Frightened. As you open your eyes and look around, nothing seems familiar. The people around you appear to be strangers.

You might have dreamt about your mother and it still feels real. You don't know that it was a dream. The past and present, dreams and reality are all merged on the same plane. You ask, "Where is my mother?"

Someone you don't recognize replies, incredulously, "Your mother is not here." You don't believe it because you were just talking to her. You feel annoyed. You want to say more but can't find the right words. You feel frustrated and angry. You think, "Don't they know that my mother is here?" You keep repeating yourself, "Where is my mother?" and someone says, "Let's wash up." For the moment, you are distracted, then upset that a stranger is trying to undress you. Later on, you ask about your mother again, but this time, no one answers you.

Finally, someone who knows how to communicate with you steps in and says, "You must miss your mother." You nod, and the person asks, "Was your mother nice to you?" You say yes, and the person asks, "Was she a good cook?"

And you start to talk, no longer upset, happy to finally have someone to speak to about what was really on your mind: your mother.

You can probably imagine the frustration and disorientation that you would feel. A person with Alzheimer's is simply not up to the task of understanding reality. This is why compassionate, empathic communication as outlined in Tool 2, Show Empathy, and using repetition, a feature of Tool 9, Use Your Loved One's Repetitions to Connect, are more effective in making a connection than changing the subject.

The Progression of Alzheimer's Disease

Alzheimer's starts slowly, progressing over a number of years. The disease can last up to twenty years, advancing from mild (early stage), to moderate (midstage), to severe (late stage). Symptoms worsen over time. Memory loss, problems with paying attention, confusion, trouble with money and finances, possible mood and personality changes, and poor judgment characterize the early stage.

Furthermore, verbal communication begins to deteriorate. The person can no longer take care of herself. Everyday activities become overwhelming. She has difficulty initiating even simple tasks. The cognitive loss affects her emotionally as well. She may report a reduced sense of self-esteem, a sense of humiliation, and a loss of control (Clare 2003).

In the middle stage, memory problems and confusion intensify. New deficits arise to create sleep disturbances, wandering, nonrecognition of family members or friends, constant repetition of ideas or statements, further deterioration in language expression, apathy, difficulties with physical movements, and restlessness. Psychotic symptoms of para-noia, delusions, or hallucination may emerge, as you may recall from chapter 9.

In the advanced stage, mental and physical deterioration continue, with a diminished capacity to produce recogniz-able words or to eat. As a rule, the disease comes to an end when the person afflicted succumbs to an infection, such as pneumonia, that overwhelms her resources to fight.

What Else May Be Going on When Talking Doesn't Work: The Quiet Ones

Sometimes people who get Alzheimer's are quiet by nature. Considering the many differences in the ways people communicate, it may be unreasonable to assume that despite your best efforts, the persistent silence of your loved one is solely a function of Alzheimer's or of depression. Perhaps he was never a big talker before. How can you expect your loved one to suddenly open up if he rarely did so in the past? The challenge becomes how to find a way to connect by using nonverbal techniques, such as touch, taste, tone, or smell, along with music, art, songs, or photographs, to supplement even successful verbal interchanges. The list *17 Ways to Promote Cooperation* in chapter 15 provides details about these approaches.

Be alert to a sudden lack of response, which may indicate that something is wrong. Use gestures, along with questions or statements that require only a yes or no answer, to deter-mine if she is in pain. Sitting too long in one position or loud noises can cause discomfort that is easily remedied. Check with other people who see your loved one regularly and find out if her nonresponsiveness is consistent. Maybe she's just having a bad day, which in itself can become the focus of a discussion.

Pain is so often underreported for people with advancing Alzheimer's and other illnesses that nursing homes and hospitals are mandated to assess everyone for pain. If you still care for your loved one at home, be sure to ask him if he is in pain, especially if he signals you with a sudden deterioration in his behavior and how he acts.

Because those with Alzheimer's have a problem with initiating conversation, acting out upsetting feelings may become their means of expression. Silence or listlessness or, at the other end of the spectrum, screaming, cursing, grimacing, or crying—all transmit the message that something is wrong, physically or emotionally.

If you cannot figure out what actually is wrong or you end up not receiving a comprehensible response, get help. A physician can assess the situation to discover what is going on medically. Behavioral upset or increased confusion are usually the first signs that your loved one is not eating properly or drinking enough fluids. A urinary tract infection or even a simple cold can trigger an uncharacteristic reaction. Note that the aging body rarely runs a fever to signal illness. When medical and physical issues have been ruled out as a cause of undue silence, consider depression, which is the focus of chapter 8.

The average duration of the disease is seven years, but Alzheimer's can linger for as long as twenty years. In the last phase, the person may be unable to speak at all. Although persistent unresponsiveness is a heartbreaker, the individual with Alzheimer's can sense if people are present. Always assume that your loved one can hear you and understand what you, or anyone else within earshot, says. The soothing tone of your voice and the gentle touch of your hand can convey love and comfort, a message that transcends barriers even if your loved one cannot respond in kind.

More About Incidence and Diagnosis

A guesstimate is that approximately one-half of the 5.3 million people in the United States who currently have Alzheimer's are in the early stages. People in the early stages may be able to explain what it is like to struggle to remember when they begin to notice that something is wrong. You may have observed this happening with someone you know.

The remaining 2.6 million are in the middle to late stages of the disease. As the disease progresses by attacking different areas of the brain, the speech and language centers falter, further interfering with expressing an idea. The ability to initiate communication is diminished or has disappeared.

Diagnosis of Alzheimer's disease is tricky. Even the experts find it a challenge because, as we have seen, many types of dementia share common symptoms, and depression or delirium can make the picture murky. At this time, there can be no absolute conclusive diagnosis of Alzheimer's while a person is alive (Mace and Rabins 2006). Nevertheless, tentative early diagnosis provides the opportunity to begin treatment so that the rate of progression will slow down and you and your loved one will have time to discuss what action to take (Marseille and Silverman 2006). After all, Alzheimer's is about a person, not just a disease.

Medical centers that offer an institute for aging or memory problems usually provide a coordinated approach to assessment and treatment, which may result in a more accurate finding. Some people worry about being stigmatized with a diagnosis of Alzheimer's. Individuals deal with this in various ways, often hiding the information from friends and family because the mere mention of Alzheimer's can trigger fear and shame. People may recoil from an individual with dementia (Smith 1992). Also, there are cultural differences in the way people view illness (Gallagher-Thompson et al. 2003). However, many of those who are open about the disease usually find support and acceptance.

A Word About Early Onset

For the approximately 5 percent of the population who develop Alzheimer's before the age of sixty-five, the disease complicates their lives and the lives of their family members even more (Peterson 2008). A person in the early-onset category may still be the primary wage earner or a caregiver of young children, so that additional financial, as well as emotional, crises may arise. Difficult issues must be addressed, including communicating with an employer, insurance carriers, children, and extended family members about the personal and financial implications of the disease (Wang 2008). The entire family structure undergoes a complete metamorphosis that intensifies the impact of the illness.

Maintaining Treatment

It is important to seek reevaluation at periodic intervals and whenever you notice a sudden change in your loved one, such as yelling, cursing, or grimacing, which may be associated with emotional or physical discomfort. Your observations about the differences in functioning and behavior provide valuable input for a medical reassessment.

After medical reevaluation, find out if your loved one should see a specialist such as a geriatrician, geropsychiatrist, neurologist, or geriatric treatment team in your area. Neuropsychological testing and a speech evaluation may pinpoint areas of strength and deficits. It takes skill and experience to sort out what is going on and to institute additional treatment.

What Else You Can Do

If you haven't already done so, get in touch with an organization such as the Alzheimer's Association or the National Alliance for Caregiving for ongoing support, understanding, and information. To find ways to restore your emotional and physical energy, see chapter 16. Continue learning more about the disease and educate your friends and family. See the Recommended Resources section at the back of the book for further details. Advocate for funding for Alzheimer's research.

If at all possible, consider enrolling yourself or your loved one in one of the many ongoing clinical studies. A shortage of research participants has been hampering research efforts. Contact the Alzheimer's Association or your local medical or university institution to explore which studies are in need of participants and which one might be best suited for your situation.

Although it is a daunting task, keep on helping your loved one to communicate by connecting his remaining but disjointed thoughts, ideas, and behavior. The rewards of making the human-to-human connection are well worth your efforts.

CHAPTER 14

More on Memory:
The Good News

How can there be good news about your loved one's severe memory loss because of Alzheimer's? Well, let's start by taking a look at memory. Memory is "the power, act, or process of recalling to mind facts previously learned or past experiences" (*Webster's New World College Dictionary* 3rd ed. 1997). It includes both the ability to acquire and retain new information, as well as retrieve past learning, experiences, and events. To learn is "to get knowledge, or skill by study, experience, instruction, etc." (*Webster's New World College Dictionary* 3rd ed. 1997). Thus, we learn material which can then be stored in our memory to be retrieved as needed.

Among the many ways of examining memory are two basic memory systems that play a significant role in Alzheimer's: explicit memory and implicit memory. *Explicit memory* is the system that encodes and retrieves information on a conscious or aware level. *Implicit memory* is the system that acquires information on an unconscious or unaware level. Explicit memory is a site of major deterioration of memory in Alzheimer's and other dementias.

The good news is that a person with mild to moderate Alzheimer's retains implicit memory, that is, the unconscious recall of information, even though she is unaware of how she learned the material (Harrison et al. 2007; Morris and Kopelman 1986). Judging from my clinical experience, it has become more apparent that implicit memory continues to work in advancing Alzheimer's as well.

These memory systems may also be called *declarative* (explicit) and *nondeclarative* or *procedural* (implicit), and they are located in separate areas of the brain (Mitchell 1988; Dick 1992; Carey 2008b). The discrete sites for these memory systems may explain why, in Alzheimer's, implicit memory partially escapes the fate of its counterpart, explicit memory, because their neural pathways are different.

Explicit Memory and Alzheimer's

Explicit memory is where we store facts and events so that we can remember them. When we are consciously aware of what we are learning, we commit the information to our memory. The way to determine what we have learned is to see whether we can recall or recognize the information we just stored in our brains by taking a conventional paper and pencil test. In early Alzheimer's, problems arise immediately in the retrieval of explicit memories, and the memory impairment continues to escalate throughout the course of the disease. You may have noticed that your loved one has trouble remembering new facts and situations.

Implicit Memory and Alzheimer's

The discovery that implicit learning continues to survive in people with Alzheimer's came from studies of individuals with amnesia and a form of dementia caused by alcohol abuse (Shimamura 1986). Individuals with Alzheimer's and other dementias can retain the ability to acquire knowledge on an unconscious level. One researcher found that those with Alzheimer's were able to learn personally relevant facts about themselves when the information was repeatedly presented to them, and that they remembered the information afterward (Arkin 1998).

Implicit memory may include remembering certain motor skills and habits because they are automatic and were imprinted in unconscious memory. For example, some people with Alzheimer's can use a toothbrush properly, which is an implicit habit, but they are unable to name it as a toothbrush or describe how they went about brushing their teeth, which are explicit skills (Harrison et al. 2007).

Being aware of the retention of implicit memory can change your perception of your loved one's comments as nonsensical: what he says actually may be rationally related to observations and experiences that register unconsciously (Sabat 2006). Recollections influence attitudes and behavior (Morris and Kopelman 1986; Sabat 2006). Practically everyone's behavior is influenced by unconscious cues; your loved one with Alzheimer's disease is no exception, as you will see in the next section.

Some Methods That Evaluate Learning

One method commonly used to assess whether a person has learned new material is to administer a test. But for individuals with Alzheimer's, the conventional paper and pencil test that measures conscious recall is an ineffective way to measure implicit learning. To assess implicit learning requires an indirect evaluation by observing "some change in performance or behavior of a person as a result of a previous experience that the person may deny or not recall having had" (Sabat 2006, p. 11). Improvement in the speed or accuracy of the task gauges whether or not implicit learning, and then memory formation, has taken place (Harrison et al. 2007).

A simple technique called a word-stem completion test, first used over twenty years ago with people who had memory deficits, pointed to the distinction between explicit and implicit recall (Morris and Kopelman 1986). An example of how this works is demonstrated when researchers give a word-stem completion test to people who have dementia. An investigator presents the participant with a list of words that includes the word "defend." Afterward, the individual's memory is tested by showing him the first three letters of the word "def___" and asking him to fill in the remaining letters. When the participant is unable to recall the word, the examiner reminds him that it had been a word on the list just given. Usually the participant replies, "What list?" The information had not registered in his explicit memory bank; he appears to have no conscious recollection of it.

However, when the examiner asks him to think of the first word that comes to mind after showing or telling him the first three letters, the respondent usually replies, "defend." Evidently, the word has been etched into his implicit or unconscious memory. This type of experiment has been repeated with comparable samples and yielded similar results (Sabat 2006; Morris and Kopelman 1986).

Research on how people with Alzheimer's process information on sensory, perceptual, and cognitive levels indicated that early-stage Alzheimer's patients did as well as healthy older adults when asked to recognize an object just by touching it (Harrison et al. 2007).

Using a different approach to measure implicit learning, another study (Mitchell 1988) employed a picture-naming task and comparison of the time needed by people with Alzheimer's to recognize a picture after seeing it once and then seeing it again, in contrast with the time needed by normal adults. The study found that people with Alzheimer's took less time to identify the same picture the second time, as did the normal adults, and that the improvement rates were the same for both groups. Repetition fostered learning.

Even people in the last stages of the disease were able to respond correctly in a picture-naming exercise, accurately naming a picture of a duck (Whall et al. 1997). Implicit memory may continue to function until the very end.

These studies suggest that those with Alzheimer's can learn and remember in an unconscious way.

Capitalizing on Implicit Learning and Memory

Some researchers have applied this new understanding of implicit memory with the hope that those with Alzheimer's will learn and maintain new skills that will improve their quality of life. In one investigation (Harrison et al. 2007), researchers devised a potential model to help people with

Alzheimer's prolong their level of basic functioning by activating and preserving implicit memories using ongoing repetition and practice.

Other investigators have identified what they believe are unconscious memory processes at work as Alzheimer's advances. Dr. Cameron Camp, an applied gerontologist, modified the Montessori approach for children to accommodate people with Alzheimer's. The Montessori method is designed for children to learn by performing certain structured tasks to develop thinking, social, and functional skills. Individuals with Alzheimer's also respond well to structure.

In one of many studies, researchers used the principles of the Montessori method in an adult day care program for people with Alzheimer's. They found that participants were significantly more interactive with each other and with their environment when compared to regular adult day care programming, citing many examples of Alzheimer's patients who were capable of unconscious learning (Judge, Camp, and Orsulic-Jeras 2000). The participants learned and retained new information, even when they couldn't remember it consciously from week to week.

Related Research

New brain cells continue to be formed for people as they age, including those with Alzheimer's (Jin et al. 2004b). Providing a rich, stimulating environment through physical and mental exercise may produce even more neurons that may foster learning (Jin et al. 2004a).

Investigators are using other approaches to see if those with early to midstage Alzheimer's can learn information that is not related to their past. In one study, researchers utilized a workbook format they entitled *Structured Practice* to see if participants could remember phone numbers after repeated drills. They found that the majority did remember some of the numbers one day later. Interestingly, the research participant who was thought to be the most cognitively impaired, according to a mental status test, was the only one who remembered the entire phone number one week later (Hochhalter, Stevens, and Okonkwo 2007).

Positive results were reported in another series of studies that focused on Alzheimer's memory training. Participants were presented personally significant factual statements, asked questions, and then given the correct answers. The examiners repeated the instructions. To their surprise, the person with the lowest score on the Mini-Mental Status Exam remembered the greatest amount of the information (Arkin 1998). In a follow-up study, most of the material was remembered for up to two months without anyone repeating the information during the interim (Arkin 2000a). Subsequently, the investigators reported comparable results in similar studies later that year (Arkin 2000b; Arkin and Mahendra 2001).

Another research project examined early-stage Alzheimer's patients who were given new material to learn and to promote conversation as they engaged in physical exercise. Caregivers stated that the social interaction had been the most beneficial aspect of the program and that overall physical stamina had increased (Arkin 2007).

Although the sample sizes were small, it would appear that people with early to midstage Alzheimer's can learn new information under certain circumstances. Perhaps by utilizing behavioral or verbal measurement, more evidence will surface to indicate that your loved one can still learn new material, even in the mid to late stages of the disease.

Implications

There is some evidence that intricate mental processes continue for those with advancing Alzheimer's, even when normal communication has ceased (Foley 1992). Moreover, it appears that one of the major emotional centers of the brain, the amygdala, may be one of the last structures to be attacked by Alzheimer's (Fleming et al. 2003; LeDoux 1993).

One study (Arkin and Mahendra 2001) determined that insight remained intact if the individual with Alzheimer's has exhibited insight previously. In some cases, insight regarding awareness of the disease actually increased over time.

Another investigation (Fleming et al. 2003) found that people with Alzheimer's exhibited better immediate recall when positive and, in particular, negative emotions were associated with the material at the time they saw it. Emotionally charged information and implicit memory may explain why a person with Alzheimer's may react negatively to people and situations he does not like, with silence, crying, screaming, or cursing. Unconsciously, he may be reminded of a perceived bad experience with that individual, and he reacts the only way he can since he can no longer use words to express what he feels. The converse may also be true: he may be happy from a previous exchange without really knowing why.

A few of the patients whom I visited were rude to people they had previously perceived as unkind or insulting; yet these same patients were friendly to those whom they sensed as kind and respectful. Somehow, much later on, they implicitly remembered their earlier impressions, even though they couldn't recall the incidents that led to those impressions.

Implicit memory may play a role in your day-to-day interactions with your loved one. Neuropsychologist Steven Sabat (2006) described how one wife began to worry about how safely her husband with Alzheimer's could mow the lawn, although mishaps had never occurred. After trying various ways to discourage her husband, she locked the woodshed door where the lawn mower was stored. But he was determined. He broke the lock, took out the lawn mower, and mowed the lawn. She then asked their son to remove the lawn mower from the shed.

When her husband went out to the woodshed the following week, he became upset because he couldn't find the lawn mower. His wife told him that their son had picked it up and was keeping it. A week later, when the son visited his parents, the father, who had always had a good relationship with his son, suddenly would not speak to him at all. Without being able to explain why, he was angry with his son. On an unconscious level, he was indignant because the son had taken the missing lawn mower. The father could not remember any part of the incident, but the emotion of anger remained in his implicit memory bank and affected his attitude.

You may be trying to determine what your loved one can and cannot do. Some skills may remain, as described in the case above, and maintaining the dignity of your loved one may call on you to swallow your apprehensions and hope for the best. Consult with a physician, physical therapist, or occupational therapist to obtain a professional recommendation.

Implicit memory may have been operating in the people I met with for individual or group therapy who were in the moderate to severe stage of Alzheimer's. Certainly, in the group, most members began to realize that something special was unfolding at every session. Expressions of recognition and delight lit up their faces whenever we all got together. Perhaps the repetition of the group sessions, the familiarity of sitting in a circle, the discussions on recurring themes, and the presence of the same group leader activated their implicit memory systems and their positive emotional associations. You can use the same tools that I used to create your own new shared memories.

This is a lesson for us all: we should approach our loved ones with Alzheimer's respectfully, being careful of what we say and how we say it. Continue your positive relationship no matter how withdrawn the person with Alzheimer's may appear to you. She may remember how special you are because of implicit memory. You can still bring joy to each other and have heartwarming moments together.

CHAPTER 15

How Do I Get My Loved One to Change? Managing Ordinary to Challenging Behavior

Normally, a person's emotional state varies throughout the day and from day to day depending upon what is happening in his life. People with Alzheimer's are no exception. How often have I started a day feeling neutral, and then I hear some good news and become elated? Later on, I run into a glitch on my computer and become frantic. Fortunately, I can understand my reactions, fix the problem, and talk to someone about my feelings if I want to. Unfortunately, those with Alzheimer's cannot do these things. Yet many relatives and caregivers want a loved one with Alzheimer's to act appropriately and to cooperate, which of course he may not be able to do consistently, and that creates tension for you both.

The way to approach challenging situations is contingent upon you changing the circumstances to foster cooperation. *You are the one who is capable of change.* The methods covered in this chapter can improve your day-to-day interactions with your loved one, as well as problem behaviors. We will look at some causes of agitated behavior, verbal and physical aggression, the condition called sundowning, and managing ordinary to challenging behavior. You will also find tips on how to promote cooperation and suggestions to improve sleep.

Causes of Agitated Behavior

Researchers report that impaired communication accounts for most of the disruptive behaviors that may arise in Alzheimer's disease (Talerico, Evans, and Strumpf 2002). When the disease advances, your loved one still has thoughts that she needs to express, and she may act out her feelings. But her actions may be insufficient to express the nuances of her feelings, and this leads to even more frustration. For example, if she is in pain, she may become cranky or shout. If she is afraid because someone is invading her privacy, she may strike out with a slap. If she is bored, she may wander, rummage through cupboards, or turn on the stove. If she feels bad because she cannot contribute to the family as she used to, she may rearrange items in drawers to feel useful. As her caregiver, you find yourself cautiously alert and you never know what to expect.

Verbal and Physical Aggression

Your loved one usually does not mean to hurt you. But frustration and anger can set off verbal or physical attacks, especially if your loved one was quick to anger in the past. Actually, cursing and yelling may indicate that he still possesses sufficient verbal resources to express irritation or rage. Research supports the contention that disruptive sounds and phrases are not devices meant just to get your attention, but rather your loved one's efforts to communicate (Matteau et al. 2003). Also, aggressive behavior may be an expression of pain. Or hitting or slapping may be a sign of rage that he can no longer control or express simply by shouting. He may hit someone as a reflexive reaction to protect himself from real or imagined danger. Sometimes, boredom can trigger emotional outbursts.

One study (Talerico, Evans, and Strumpf 2002) found a strong relationship between depression and physical aggression and conjectured that aggression may be a sign of inadequately treated depression. Once again, a sudden onset of any of the symptoms discussed above calls for an expert to rule out medical or emotional illness.

Researchers have pointed out that direct treatment of aggression with the use of antipsychotic medications often produces negative side effects, such as an increase in confusion, unsteadiness in using one's hands or walking, sleepiness, weight gain, and increased risk of stroke (Sink, Holden, and Yaffe 2005). Furthermore, the medications have limited impact on reducing aggressive behavior. The pharmaceutical approach may not be the answer for treating an agitated loved one (Schneider et al. 2006; Sink, Holden, and Yaffe 2005). However, further on in this chapter you will read about methods that can target underlying needs such as sensory deprivation, boredom, or loneliness and may ease the burden and reduce physical or emotional outbursts (Cohen-Mansfield 2001).

Sundowning

Your loved one may be among the approximately 25 percent of those with Alzheimer's who become more confused later in the day, an occurrence known as *sundowning* (Taylor et al. 1997). As the sun begins to descend on the horizon, your loved one may literally become more addled, restless, suspicious, demanding, and unruly. She may yell, pace, strike out, or even hallucinate, thus creating serious problems for caregivers. You too may have become more exhausted by the end of the day, and it may take great effort for both of you to keep it together. However, the person with Alzheimer's has even less wherewithal to make it through the day without deteriorating. The following morning, he will be calmer and wake up the way he usually does, with little evidence of the behavior you witnessed the previous afternoon or evening. Note that if you want to stimulate conversation to connect more meaningfully, plan to have those discussions earlier in the day, before fatigue sets in.

The good thing about sundowning is that it is predictable. That means you can have a plan for what to do during those late afternoon to early evening hours, before the symptoms appear. You may have to start with a look at his sleep patterns, since irregular sleep patterns contribute to sundowning. As you read on, apply the suggestions listed in managing behaviors, in addition to the approaches that follow later on about how to deal with sleep disturbances.

How to Manage Ordinary to Challenging Behavior

Whether your loved one is generally compliant or not, she is incapable of changing her behavior. The responsibility for managing the situation falls exclusively on your shoulders or those of other caregivers.

The key to dealing with ordinary and challenging behavior lies in understanding the meaning of the behavior. Then you can modify the dynamics of the situation. You need to determine what is causing the upset or the aggressive behavior. This task may be even more daunting than looking for meaning in fragmented phrases can be. You must have patience and pay close attention to what is going on. Remember that if she could tell you directly what was bothering her, she probably would.

First, identify exactly what the problem is. Think back to what happened just before the incident. Who was with your loved one at that time? What was going on? At what time of day did the incident occur? What could possibly have set her off? Could her reaction have been motivated by what someone else did? Check with whoever was providing care at that time, because your loved one may not remember the incident.

Then take a look at what happened afterward. What did your loved one do? What did you do? Jot down what occurred after the outburst subsided, including your own feelings and reactions. Carefully observe and keep a written record of what you see.

Examine your notes and look for any patterns that catch your eye. Did any flare-ups occur at the same time of day or during the same kind of activity? Are other people usually present at that time, and are they usually the same people? Was the same activity going on before each outburst? Were there background noises or other distractions? Did someone yell at her? Was she criticized or called names?

Put it all together to find the meaning of her behavior. When you succeed in figuring out what set off her reaction, you can then modify circumstances in advance to deflect the negative response. If the cause was unavoidable, such as providing morning care that your loved one perceived as a stranger undressing her, have a plan that can defuse the situation, such as involving your loved one in the care process so that she participates while you softly explain every single step of what you are doing. Here are some general guidelines that will promote cooperative behaviors.

17 Ways to Promote Cooperation

1. Stay calm, especially if there is a crisis.

2. Avoid using negatives and "don'ts."

3. If the behavior erupts at a certain time of day, anticipate the difficult time and be especially reassuring in a soft, gentle way before and after that time.

4. Ask her if it's all right to place your hand on her arm or shoulder, and be sure to be gentle.

5. Have your loved one participate in personal care. For example, give her a washcloth to clean herself as you use a washcloth to clean her. Or place your hand on hers and gently guide her. Be soothing and reassuring. Explain everything you are doing as you do it.

6. Prior to the time of day he may become agitated, gently guide your loved one into an activity by saying, "Please come with me...," instead of, "Would you like to come with me?" which could invite a refusal.

7. Engage in simple physical exercise such as a walk outside, dancing to music, or tossing a ball. One study (Teri et al. 2003) found a significant improvement in physical functioning and a reduction in depression in Alzheimer's patients still living at home when caregivers oversaw a practice of exercise combined with behavioral management. Another study (Arkin 2003) noted that physical exercise produced an increase in physical fitness and mood for Alzheimer's patients who did not have problems with aggression. A stroll together out of doors can do wonders for anyone's disposition and channel the excess energy that can fuel outbursts or unsupervised wandering behavior.

8. Initiate an activity such as playing soft music (Alzheimer's Association 2006), engaging in a simple art project, gardening, playing cards, or anything else you know that she usually enjoys. Consider reading aloud from a newspaper, a book, or a poem that would interest her.

9. Plan to sing together prior to a potential upset, or just to have some fun together, to reinforce interaction and promote relaxation (Clair 2002; Clair, Matthews, and Kosloski 2005).

10. Offer her a stuffed animal or a soft blanket if she would find that reassuring. The tactile sense of touch can be very soothing.

11. Consider animal therapy with a gentle or specially trained animal, such as a rabbit or dog, for your loved one to pet. The research literature reports promising findings that using this approach may reduce agitation in your loved one regardless of the progression of the disease (Richeson 2003).

12. Use prayer or song if either usually comforts your loved one.

13. Use lemon or lavender oil, even though her sense of smell has diminished. Inhaling certain agents in these oils calms the brain, as will massaging a diluted form of the oil into the skin (Cawthorn 1995; Worwood and Worwood 2003).

14. Reduce environmental stimuli by turning off loud radios and TVs and eliminating loud or distracting conversations going on around her.

15. Always explain each step of what you do in a soft, reassuring way.

16. Allow a few minutes for her to respond to what you have tried.

17. Continue to follow a set routine every day to minimize confusion and foster trust.

For people in long-term care facilities, as well as at home, techniques such as personalizing space and using cues associated with their routines when they were younger often help them remember. For example, you could place a photograph of a toothbrush, sink, and toilet on the door of the bathroom, a picture of a bed on the door of the bedroom, and pictures of food, plates, and silverware on the door of the kitchen. The cue could be a picture of your loved one washing up or eating. Conversely, do not identify places you would prefer he not go, such as the front door or closets.

If you need more help with learning how to apply these suggestions, contact a local organization such as the Alzheimer's Association or the National Family Caregivers Association, both of which offer classes and conferences and provide literature about many aspects of Alzheimer's care. See the Recommended Resources at the back of the book.

If aggressive outbursts persist, seek a geriatric medical specialist who may recommend medication (Sink, Holden, and Yaffe 2005). Make sure to find out how this treatment may help. As an astute consumer, ask the physician to tell you about the use of herbal medicines that may alleviate agitation. Herbs such as *Melissa officinalis* (lemon balm) and *Salvia officinalis* (sage) may be recommended as an adjunct to the treatment plan (Akhondzadeh and Abbasi 2006). A word to the wise: avoid administering any herbal supplements, which are actually drugs, without the expressed approval of your physician.

Sleep Disturbances

Sleep disorders affect many people with Alzheimer's, as well as their caregivers. Your loved one's sleeping patterns will create disturbances for you as well. Furthermore, any kind of disruptive behavior may be related to a problem with falling asleep and staying asleep throughout the night. Surprisingly, the more a person with Alzheimer's sleeps, including frequent daytime napping and going to bed early at night, the more aggressive that person is during the day, with wandering during the night (Ancoli-Israel et al. 2004). Moreover, "going to bed early and increased use of sedative hypnotics [sleep medications] were associated with caregiver reports of increased wandering at night and more aggressive behavior during the day" (Taylor et al. 1997, p. 116). As stated earlier, sleep irregularities contribute to the problems of sundowning, so any improvement in the sleep cycle may alleviate late afternoon agitation.

Limiting daytime naps to only one a day, for no more than an hour in the early afternoon, and delaying bedtime for your loved one may help. A consistent short nap, not more than one hour in the early afternoon, can actually assist in new memory formation (Tucker and Fishbein 2008).

One nursing facility, the Hebrew Home at Riverdale in New York, instituted a novel approach to deal with day-night reversal. They formulated a full, stimulating program all night long for those who were up at night and asleep during the day (Buckley 2009).

There is always treatment with medication, which may have many undesirable side effects, including increased confusion, and it may not improve sleep (Dowling 1996). Tackle the sleeping problem initially by instituting some basic practices that may promote good sleeping habits. Disruptive sleep patterns can be the final contributing factor for a caregiver to decide to place a loved one in a long-term care facility. The following suggestions may improve the situation.

9 Ways to Improve Sleep

1. Expose your loved one to light late in the day. Sitting in afternoon sunlight, even for thirty to forty-five minutes, may help. Getting some daylight at the end of a day improves sleep at night (Ancoli-Israel 2004; Dowling 1996).

2. Maximize daytime physical activity. Do some kind of exercise, from as little as six minutes to thirty minutes a few times per week, or as much as your loved one can tolerate (Dowling 1996).

3. Provide your loved one with heat, such as giving him a warm bath, toward the end of the day (Dowling 1996).

4. Minimize daytime napping. If she naps, make sure it is only once a day, in the early afternoon, and at the same time each day (Dowling 1996).

5. In general, restrict time spent in bed during the day (Dowling 1996).

6. Do not let your loved one ingest any caffeine (coffee, chocolate, or cola drinks) after 12 noon.

7. Restrict fluid intake after 6 in the evening.

8. Make sure he avoids all alcohol, since alcohol contributes to waking up after a few hours of sleep.

9. Make sure your loved one has a consistent bedtime routine, going to bed at the same time every night.

Here's to a good night's sleep for you both.

CHAPTER 16

How About You? Care for the Caregiver

Who are your fellow travelers also taking the journey through Alzheimer's with a loved one? You and your relatives and friends are among the estimated 10 million unpaid caregivers, not to mention the many paid caregivers in nursing homes or long-term care facilities. You have a lot of company.

Here are some statistics:

- Approximately 70 percent of the people with dementia live at home and are cared for by family members and friends (Alzheimer's Association 2009, p. 15). The largest clusters of caregivers are spouses, followed by daughters and daughters-in-law. Sons account for the smallest number: 6 percent (Montgomery and Kosloski 2002). Grandchildren, nieces, and nephews contribute care as well.

- Although the percentage varies from study to study, caregivers are mainly women, who are estimated to do over 70 percent of the caregiving (Montgomery and Kosloski 2002), although recent trends reported by the National Alliance for Caregiving and the Alzheimer's Association indicate a dramatic increase in the number of males who assist with the care of a relative with any kind of illness (Leland 2008). These figures are based on the numbers of people who contribute in any way to the care of a loved one.

- Women, as the primary caregivers, bear the brunt of the job. In addition to their other responsibilities, primary caregivers devote an average of 16 to as much as 40 hours a week to caregiving, in addition to employment and other household responsibilities. Typically, the vast majority of dementia caregivers experience emotional stress reactions such as frustration and exhaustion.

- The financial impact of caring for someone with Alzheimer's is huge. In the United States, the Alzheimer's Association estimates the overall cost as $148 billion annually (Alzheimer's Association 2009). By 2010, the cost is expected to be over $160 billion (Alzheimer's Association 2007). Family members pay for most of the expenditures for care, with large out-of-pocket expenses in addition to what's covered by medical insurance. In 2006, the average salaries of home health aides were $19 an hour (Alzheimer's Association 2007). Adult day care services were $64 per day, and nursing home care approximately $75,000 annually (Alzheimer's Association 2009).

Caregivers come from every culture, and each culture has its own traditions about how to care for loved ones who are ill. As you read on, some suggestions may be more comfortable for you than others. Choose whatever feels right for you. The following subjects are covered in this chapter: what it means to be a caregiver, caregiver stress, how to find relief, and sixteen ways to care for yourself.

What It Means to Be a Caregiver

To be a *caregiver* is to help someone who is unable to take care of herself. Caregiving, to some extent, is a normal part of all relationships; it is a heartfelt manifestation of one's dedication to the welfare of another (Pearlin et al. 1990). Some people experience caregiving as a truly spiritual experience, while other caregivers see it as a burden. Overseeing the care of your spouse, partner, or parent can be an on-site, day and night responsibility when your loved one lives at home.

Caregivers can fall into one of two categories: primary or secondary. If you are the *primary caregiver*, you oversee all of the personal, logistical, and emotional needs of your loved one. This can be a full-time job. If you are a *secondary caregiver*, you fill in and do fewer tasks for shorter periods of time. You may research options for care or handle financial concerns. You may volunteer to help out with physical tasks or you may work as a paid aide. If you live some distance away from your loved one and have a relative who has assumed the role of primary caregiver, you may fulfill some of these functions and provide support.

Caregiving in Couples

When Alzheimer's descends upon one member of a couple, the other member often assumes responsibility as the primary caregiver. As a result, the balance of responsibility and position in the larger family unit shift, and both you and your loved one undergo radical transformation in your relationship with each other.

The arrival of Alzheimer's shatters the dream couples have of aging together, of spending their golden years together with no job pressures or traveling to places they've always wanted to see. If you are among the younger couples who face early-onset Alzheimer's, complicated, thorny issues arise, such as how to provide for a young family financially and emotionally. Regardless of age, when one partner becomes the person in need, no longer able to provide or relate as was done earlier in the relationship, both partners undergo radical shifts in their identities.

Now one provides direct care for the physical needs of the other or makes arrangements for paid care. A wife may find herself the new financial manager, suddenly in charge of paying bills, writing checks, and submitting medical claims, all of which may be duties that her husband used to perform. A husband may find himself having to learn how to prepare meals, do laundry, become a social secretary, or coordinate schedules. Economic pressures mount. Emotional strains take their toll. You may feel cheated. You may feel resentful.

Impact on Children and Friends

Even when family interactions had been smooth, conflict may arise among various family members who express different approaches to the care of your loved one. Note that if conflict was a part of family dynamics prior to onset of the disease, disagreement is more likely to occur afterward.

Children and friends watch the transition with sadness and dread. They may find themselves facing the confusion of a role reversal in their parent-child relationship or the friend-to-friend tie, as the loved one can no longer be turned to for help or advice. Adult daughters may take on a dominant role as they struggle to balance the needs of their own families with the needs of a parent. Younger children have multiple needs to be met as they face the prospect of losing a parent to early-onset Alzheimer's or a beloved grandparent to the onslaught of the disease.

Yet your loved one is certainly not a child, despite her progressive loss of functioning. She is very much an individual who is battling a disease that robs her of the ability to take care of herself and be herself.

Grieving the Loss

Everyone, including your loved one, begins a kind of grieving for the loss of the person you both knew and the loss of your life together before the disease struck (Dempsey and Baago 1998). This grief may cause you to let go of your loved one prematurely just as he struggles to hold on to himself. Emotions churn as the grief process proceeds. You may long for the person who used to be, and you may feel anger and sadness as you continue to bear witness to the losses that Alzheimer's imposes on your loved one and yourself.

Caregiver Stress: Hidden Victims and Hidden Heroes

Stress is the mental and physical tension created by strain. You carry an enormous burden of responsibility that adds to your own stress as your loved one becomes more and more dependent on your assistance to carry out basic functions. As you oversee the actions of your loved one, you may become hypervigilant, which may increase stress. Communication impairments such as repetitive questioning and the inability to communicate either verbally or nonverbally serve to make your responsibilities even harder. You may worry about what comes next. Just when you adjust to one routine, another loss usually presents itself, so that you must alter your routine to integrate the new problem.

In a way, you become the hidden victim of this disease, as well as the hidden hero, as you tirelessly give of yourself, often neglecting your own basic human needs. You do the very best you can in providing care. It is a testimony to how much your loved one means to you. Furthermore, if you are a primary caregiver, you make up the schedules, set appointments, assign duties to the secondary caregivers, and oversee all of the necessities of your loved one.

Whether you give care directly or through a hired helper, anxiety and depression may settle in. One group of researchers noted, "Dementia caregivers commonly experience elevated levels of stress, and are at increased risk for psychological disorders" (Spira et al. 2007 p. 56). You may feel resentment because you may assume that your loved one's challenging behavior is a ploy to control you when, in fact, he has no control over the way Alzheimer's attacks him. Paid caregivers undergo similar issues, but they have the advantage of knowing that caregiving is a job they have chosen, and they can go home to their own lives at the end of the shift.

Interestingly, in studies of caregiver stress, the way you look at what is happening to you and your loved one profoundly affects how well you cope. For example, in studies of couples, those caregivers who saw the situation as a continuation of their connection with their loved one fared better with coping. They also interacted more with their loved ones than those who reacted mainly to the negative changes in their partner (Lewis et al. 2005).

Stress can have a negative impact on your physical health as well (Alzheimer's Association 2009). Make sure that you do not neglect your own annual medical and dental checkups, and remember to keep healthy snacks such as fruits, nuts, and vegetables on hand (Brody 2008).

Caregiving does not end if you place your loved one in a nursing facility. You may feel overwhelming guilt and sadness along with relief (Lichtenberg 2006), and your responsibilities continue even though they shift to visitations and advocacy for the best care possible. Taking care of yourself is still as important as it was when your loved one lived at home.

You Are Not Alone: Ways to Find Relief

When you become so involved in the care of another, it is easy to lose yourself and not realize the toll it takes on you. In the last stages of Alzheimer's, care for a loved one at home occupies practically all of the caregiver's free time (Aguglia et al. 2004).

Isolation plays a significant role in Alzheimer's. Not only is your loved one isolated as the disease causes her to withdraw, but you can also become isolated as social engagements dwindle and people stop visiting. Any measures you can take to reduce the isolation can be of value to you both. That's why it is so crucial for you to pay attention to yourself by building in time for yourself in your busy schedule of providing care.

Taking Care of Yourself

You could use a break from the ongoing care you give to your loved one. In order to take care of yourself, you will need some help from others. By facing this fact early on, before your loved one requires even more extensive assistance, you provide yourself with an opportunity to explore your options and to bring in some helpers for you and your loved one to get to know.

You could use some support. Support is defined as a series of connections on physical, emotional, and socially interactive levels that will give you some relief from the burdens you face. Support can be as basic as someone coming by to take a turn staying with your loved one while you do something else. Or it could be the comfort and understanding you receive from talking to someone who is going through a similar situation.

Research indicates that having someone with whom you can confide on a regular basis reduces the stress of caregiving (Gaugler et al. 2004). Study after study suggests that the stronger your support system is, the better you will feel and the healthier you will be. Results show that those who care for people with Alzheimer's are healthier when they receive support from others in the same situation (Spira et al. 2007).

Sometimes family members find it hard to accept help from others. Your loved one with Alzheimer's may be possessive of you as the one she still recognizes and you may feel guilty when you have the opportunity to take a break. Or you may feel that there is no one else to turn to. Yet if you don't take time for yourself, you put your own mental and physical well-being in jeopardy.

There is plenty of support available if you know how to access it. Here are some ideas.

16 Self-Care Tools for You

1. **General support groups.** Support groups usually consist of a small cluster of caregivers who meet with a trained leader to discuss various topics related to a common issue, in this case, caring for people with Alzheimer's. Participants report an increase in coping skills when they attend psychoeducational groups that provide salient information about the disease (Onor et al. 2007). The interactions and the sharing among members are invaluable. You help each other through the simple act of conversing—saying what it is really like and hearing others describe what it is really like for them. You offer solutions to common problems and learn new ways to deal with challenges. Laughter and tears mix with frustration and anger. If you live in an urban or suburban area, support groups such as those sponsored by the Alzheimer's Association abound. These kinds of groups have sprung up all over the United States and around the world.

2. **Support groups for partners or spouses.** Marriages can become destabilized once Alzheimer's is diagnosed (Lichtenberg 2006). Nonetheless, researchers have found that participation in a couples group was a positive experience for couples consisting of one partner who was the caregiver and the other who had Alzheimer's (Logsdon, McCurry, and Teri 2006).

3. **Support groups for those in the early stages of the disease.** Not only do the participants with Alzheimer's learn about the disease and process their own reactions, but caregivers have free time while their loved ones are meeting.

4. **Adult day care programs.** Contact your local senior citizen center. Needs of those in the early to mid stages of Alzheimer's may be met by an adult day care program staffed with professionals who know how to stimulate and interest your loved one. You, in turn, gain some time for yourself.

5. **One-to-one support.** Some people do not feel comfortable participating in small groups. A few of the organizations listed below (see item 14 in this list) may have people available for private one-to-one sessions.

6. **Have a friend or relative lend you a hand.** A friend, niece, nephew, cousin, or grandchild may be glad to help you and happy to have the opportunity to connect with your loved one. Arranging for someone else to take over daily, even if only for an hour, so

that you can take a walk, run an errand, or have coffee with a friend would be good for you.

7. **Telephone contact.** Some communities have set up telephone hotlines for caregivers to talk with a buddy or join in conference calls, especially in more rural areas where 27 percent of all family caregivers reside (Dollinger, Chwalisz, and Zerth 2006).

8. **Internet.** Chat rooms, blogs, and websites of various organizations can reduce your isolation and offer tips on providing care. They are usually free services.

9. **Local place of worship.** Reaching out to your local clergyperson can link you with assistance for meals and other services, as well as providing you with someone with whom you can speak in confidence.

10. **A visiting nurse or home health aide.** A visiting nurse or home health aide can stop by and help out by providing direct care. Check with the Visiting Nurse Association in your area, local newspapers, or home health care agencies.

11. **Exercise alone or with others.** Physical exercise is essential for your health and your brain. Exercise reduces stress and improves your sleep (King et al. 2002).

12. **Continue to engage in the activities you enjoy.** Engaging in the activities you have always enjoyed, healthy eating, and mental stimulation are essential for nourishing your brain, as well as your body, and will

keep you interested in life. Get some rest and relaxation. Have fun. Laugh with friends.

13. **Respite care.** This is a category all its own. *Respite care* describes any kind of assistance you receive in providing for your loved one's needs. This can include a short nursing home stay for your loved one so that you can take some time off. Consider contacting a local nursing facility to place your loved one for a weekend, if no one else can spare the time to pitch in, so that you can obtain a much-needed break for yourself. Many local nursing facilities offer this option and you can present your weekend away as an opportunity for your loved one with Alzheimer's to have a break from you, as well. Extend reassurance that you will soon be back and arrange for other relatives or friends to visit while you are away. Studies have shown that caregivers who avail themselves of respite care delay nursing home placement for their loved ones (Kosloski and Montgomery 1995) and find relief from stress.

14. **Contact an organization.** The Alzheimer's Association, the National Alliance for Caregiving, and the National Aging Information Center are among the national organizations you can get in touch with for the locations of their local branches, information, fact sheets, suggestions, support groups, individual help, and advocacy. You can download appropriate literature. Check with your local medical providers for information about programs and providers of services. A local college or university can also

provide valuable leads. Take the leap, contact one of these organizations, and join a group.

15. **Look for community support.** Local senior citizen centers may have a cadre of volunteers willing to help you with meals, shopping, and other chores. Some communities are beginning to organize volunteers to assist all caregivers and provide relief by offering free services. You owe it to yourself to check out what your community has to offer.

16. **See the recommended resources section in the back of this book for more details on how to find help.**

As a caregiver, you are engaged in a noble task that requires the courage and flexibility to connect with the essence of your loved one while preserving yourself. *You may continue to be a caregiver for quite some time, so you owe it to yourself to make the time to take care of yourself.*

CHAPTER 17

I Have a Voice Inside:
A Note of Thanks

Interviews with people in the middle stages of dementia indicate that a sense of self prevails throughout the course of the disease when the people who interact with them respond to and treat them with respect and dignity. Apparently, the person with dementia is not only capable of experiencing a sense of self, but can grow and develop when someone is sensitive to how she feels (Holst and Hallberg 2003). Even people with poor ability to think have been able to describe how they feel about having dementia (Ostwald, Duggleby, and Hepburn 2002). Remember that your loved one may still have insight, if having insight is characteristic of how she always has been (Arkin and Mahendra 2001).

A study on how caregivers approach those with Alzheimer's suggested that a person with the disease perceives patronizing speech as uncaring, disrespectful, and controlling (Small,

Perry, and Lewis 2005). Your loved one is not a child, even though she needs so much assistance to survive.

It is even more important to recognize what your loved one can do, rather than to always focus on what he cannot do (Foley 1992). The following features may persist despite the progression of the disease:

- He may draw on the social skills he used throughout his life, saying "hello," "thank you," "you're welcome," and "please." These are words he may continue to remember, in a genuine way, to make a connection (Edelson and Lyons 1985).

- She appreciates being included in conversations.

- He is grateful to participate in any activity he can contribute to. This enhances his self-image and maintains his dignity.

- She probably has the ability to acquire information through an unconscious memory process.

- He can usually tell the difference between the "good guys" and the "bad guys."

- She may be reliving an experience based on fragments of ideas that keep catching her attention.

- He has snippets of memories of other people in his life, and of celebrations or losses, past or present.

- She is grateful that you listen to her.

- He may have spiritual needs that transcend the conscious mind.

- She displays behavior that signals what she cannot say, but what she is feeling (Edelson and Lyons 1985).

- He is aware of the nature of his surroundings, even though he may not know where he is. He knows when it is noisy, quiet, light, or dark, if music is playing, and whether the air is fresh or stale.

- She uses gestures, facial expressions, eyes, touch, sound, and body position to communicate when she can no longer use words or understood them, and she realizes that you are using these ways of communicating, too.

By now you know that you and your loved one can stay connected and share precious moments together despite the ravages of Alzheimer's disease. By now you know that your loved one continues to have the emotional capacity to laugh or cry, to feel affirmed or shamed, to be funny or humorless, to be compassionate or selfish, to be happy or sad, to be fun loving or lonely, and to know love.

By now you know that your loved one has a great sense of appreciation for all that you do, and for keeping communication alive, even if she's unable to say so.

Thank you for understanding that I love you even though
I cannot remember your name or exactly who you are.
Thank you for caring for me in such a loving way.
Thank you for reaching out to me, for connecting the dots
of what I say, even though I seem like I don't want you to.

The Tools: A Summary

Here is a list that summarizes the tools. The second list repeats each tool with related comments. The first six tools are the basis for any connection with a person who has Alzheimer's disease.

Brief Summary of Tools

1. Attitude—Treat Your Loved One as a Precious Human Being

2. Show Empathy

3. Use What You Know to Go with the Flow

4. Agree

5. Have Hope and Express Love

6. Make Sure You Can Be Heard and Seen

28. Consider Your Loved One's Native Language

29. Be Prepared for Nonrecognition

30. Expect That Some Things Are Remembered

31. Learn from Your Loved One

32. Let Her Do What She Still Can Do

33. Do Not Underestimate Feelings About Saying Good-Bye

The Tools with Related Comments

Tool 1: Attitude—Treat Your Loved One as a Precious Human Being

- Smile.

- Always introduce yourself and greet your loved one by name every time you meet.

- Position yourself face-to-face or catty-corner on the same physical plane to establish eye contact.

- Use an inviting tone.

- Be kind.

- Be considerate.

- Speak slowly.

- Use gestures as you speak.

- Ask simple but open-ended questions.

- Be patient. Allow time for responses.

- Believe that your efforts may pay off.

Tool 2: Show Empathy

- Put yourself in her shoes to figure out what she may be thinking and feeling.

- Use your intuition about what you think she is saying and feeling. Connect the fragments and see if she agrees.

- Remember that your loved one is a person with dementia, not a demented person.

- Listen.

Tool 3: Use What You Know to Go with the Flow

- Use what you know about the person to understand what is being said.

- Acknowledge his reality by repeating his statement back to him and expanding on what he said.

- Go with the flow of your loved one's remarks by following up on what he said.

- Talk about memories from a long time ago since they are the last to fade.

- Don't expect him to remember your previous conversation.

- Remember that he lives in the present moment.

- View each time you meet as an entirely new occasion.

Tool 4: Agree

- Don't disagree or argue.

- Acknowledge the thoughts and feelings behind the message.

- Validate what you hear.

Tool 5: Have Hope and Express Love

- Express love and support as often as possible and your loved one may reciprocate.

- Focus on what remains, not what is gone.

- Accept her as she is.

Tool 6: Make Sure You Can Be Heard and Seen

- Always have a hearing amplifier with you, even if your loved one refuses to wear it. An amplifier can be purchased at a general electronics store.

- Reoffer the use of a hearing amplifier every time you want to communicate.

- Be prepared to repeat what you say and, if you are not alone, what others say.

- Place yourself eye to eye so that you can be seen.

Tool 7: Don't Take an Unkind Remark Too Seriously

- Have a sense of humor even when insensitive, possibly true, remarks are made.

- Try not to take it personally, even though the comments might hurt. If you feel very hurt, let him know by simply saying something like, "Ouch. That hurt."

Tool 8: Be Open

- Expect your loved one's mood to change without any warning, and don't be dismayed when this happens.

- Assume he understands, have no expectations that he will respond, and you may be pleasantly surprised.

Tool 9: Use Your Loved One's Repetitions to Connect

- Constant repetition is an opportunity to communicate.

- Delve beneath the statements to find meaning.

- Ask her opinion about any issue that is brought up.

- Connect the fragments to help her express herself.

Tool 10: Deal with Accusations

- Acknowledge that an item is not there or validate his perception that something is wrong. Be sympathetic.

- Offer to help find what is missing or to straighten out the situation.

- Apologize if your loved one says that you did something wrong.

- Once again, don't take it personally.

Tool 11: Use Foods to Awaken Memory

■ Offer your loved one a favorite food or a nonalcoholic drink.

■ Use food as a springboard to awaken memory and pleasant sensations.

Tool 12: Some Openers to Use with Men

■ Introduce news about sports or other current events as a way to communicate.

■ Again, restate what you hear.

■ Listen to a joke and laugh, no matter many times you've heard it before.

■ A sense of humor endures for a long time. Have fun laughing together.

Tool 13: Acknowledge Loss

■ Acknowledge and discuss any kind of loss.

■ Talk about your loved one's parents in order to stimulate conversation and promote healing, asking questions such as, "What was your mother like?"

■ Acknowledge and explore feelings, even the sad ones, whether or not he realizes that the relative is gone.

Tool 14: Use Meaningful Photographs to Relate

■ Use photographs and make comments to stimulate memory and to relate.

- Say something about the photograph.

- Explore your loved one's responses.

Tool 15: Use Art as a Way to Relate

- Create art with your loved one to inspire self-expression and connection.

- Discuss the meaning of what you both produce.

- Elicit your loved one's opinion about a painting you both view and ask, "What do you think of it?" Or you can ask, "What do you think it is saying?"

Tool 16: Use Singing and Music to Connect

- Music is a wonderful way to cross the barriers of isolation.

- Music can communicate beyond words alone.

- Be courageous and sing along. It's fun!

Tool 17: Set Up the Same Seating Location to Jog Memory

- Establish a regular seating arrangement each time you sit down to relate.

- Using the same seating configuration may improve your loved one's ability to recognize people and places.

Tool 18: Use Prayer if It's Appropriate

- Praying can be a healing experience. Acknowledge prayer.

- Use prayer if it's appropriate for you or your loved one.

- Living in the moment is the reality for you and your loved one.

Tool 19: There's Not Always a Simple Answer for a Change in Attitude

- Your loved one may make mean remarks.

- You can't expect your loved one to be reasonable.

- Accept her limitations.

- Your loved one may not respond to any approach.

- No one has all the answers for someone's behavior.

- Change the environment since your loved one cannot change.

- Don't take it personally.

- Find support from others who know what it's like and share your feelings.

Tool 20: Be Persistent but Respectful

- It takes time for someone with Alzheimer's to sense that you are a friendly face.

- Respect a response of no, but ask again later.

- Sharing silence is a way to connect.

Tool 21: Assume That Your Loved One Can Understand

- Assume that people are reachable even if they seem uninterested or withdrawn. Don't give up. Keep using the tools.

- Offer choices, issue invitations, not demands, and support participation.

- Your loved one may understand or remember more than you may think.

Tool 22: Check for Signs of Depression

- Observe whether your loved one is changing for the worse.

- Ask your loved one about feeling sad and be ready to discuss it.

- Have a professional assess for depression or illness.

Tool 23: Avoid Confrontation

- Avoid confrontation. Again, do not argue.

- Be empathic with your loved one who may be unable to recognize his limitations.

- Acknowledge his reality by saying that as hard as it is to believe, everyone is only trying to help. When he says that he doesn't need help, simply nod in agreement and say, "I know, I know."

Tool 24: Use the Delusion

- Interact with your loved one about the delusional material she expresses.

- See the delusion as an expression of thoughts and wishes.

- Explore a delusion as you would for any fragments you hear.

- Accept the delusion as part of her reality.

Tool 25: Self-Image Counts

- Realize that her appearance may still be important to her.

- Involve your loved one in choosing what to wear.

- Offer an either-or choice to simplify decision making.

- Compliment her to support her selection. Enjoy the experience.

Tool 26: Capitalize on Remaining Social Skills

- Basic social amenities such as "hello," "how are you," and "thank you" are bridges for either of you to connect.

- Keep on interacting even if he doesn't make much sense.

Tool 27: Be Reassuring

- It is important to acknowledge, respect, and address her concerns, whatever the situation.

- Reassurance can reduce anxiety and induce cooperation.

Tool 28: Consider Your Loved One's Native Language

- Your loved one may remember and understand communication in his native language rather than English.

- Your loved one may have difficulty understanding English that is spoken with an accent.

Tool 29: Be Prepared for Nonrecognition

- Be prepared for your loved one to forget your name or who you are.

- Understand that this loss of memory is beyond his control.

- He may still remember someone important to him.

Tool 30: Expect That Some Things Are Remembered

- Your loved one may remember an event that has a strong emotional association.

- A coherent retelling occasionally may arise.

Tool 31: Learn from Your Loved One

- Listen and learn.

- Find ways to help your loved one feel useful.

Tool 32: Let Her Do What She Still Can Do

- After consulting with an expert, permit your loved one to do what she still is capable of doing, even if it's nerve-racking for you to watch.

- Oversee the task.

- Give her time to accomplish the task. Be patient.

- Be aware of your own feelings and think before you act.

Tool 33: Do Not Underestimate Feelings About Saying Good-Bye

- He has feelings about you leaving, and so do you.

- Let him know that you will be leaving. First tell him 10 minutes before leaving, and then 5 minutes before you go.

- He recognizes and appreciates kindness.

- Accept his feelings.

Glossary of Terms

Agnosia: a sensory impairment in the ability to recognize familiar objects.

Alzheimer's disease: a progressive, degenerative, and irreversible dementia that eventually affects every aspect of the individual's personality, health, lifestyle, and relationships.

Aphasia: a language or speech-processing deficit.

Caregiver: anyone who provides help to a person who is partially to completely unable to take care of himself.

Communication: the process of transmitting information from one person to another.

Connection: a binding together; a joining between two human beings.

Delirium: a condition of mental confusion that may include delusions and hallucinations.

Delusion: a fixed belief held by someone even though there is no evidence that the belief is true.

Dementia: an impairment of memory, intellect, judgment, and emotional functioning.

Depression: an emotional state of despondency that involves feelings of hopelessness and inadequacy.

Explicit memory: the system of remembering on a conscious level.

Hallucination: a false perception of something that an individual believes she actually sees, hears, or smells, and is real to her, but is not actually present.

Implicit memory: the system of remembering on an unconscious level.

Memory: the ability to acquire and retain knowledge or learned information about experiences or past events and to retrieve this information.

Mild cognitive impairment: a memory deficit that does not interfere with daily functioning.

Neuron: a nerve cell body located in the brain and nervous system.

Paranoia: a delusion in which a person becomes irrationally suspicious and believes that someone is going to harm him.

Perseveration: the incessant repetition of certain phrases or ideas.

Spirituality: the manifestation of a life-giving force; the soul, as distinguished from the corporeal, or the body.

Recommended Resources

Internet Resources

Organizations with Comprehensive Information in the U.S.

Alzheimer's Association
800-272-3900
www.alz.org

The 24-hour hotline answers calls seven days a week to serve people with memory loss, caregivers, and professionals. The website has many resources, including message boards for people with Alzheimer's and early-onset dementia, chat rooms, and information in Spanish and other languages, as well as comprehensive fact sheets concerning all aspects of Alzheimer's and caregiving.

Alzheimer's Disease Education and Referral Center
800-438-4380
www.nia.nih.gov/Alzheimer's

This U.S. government website sponsored by the National Institute on Aging provides health information including abstracts, pamphlets, and publications.

Alzheimer's Foundation of America
866-232-8484
www.alzfdn.org

The website of this service organization includes comprehensive information on all aspects of Alzheimer's disease. Their Care Connection offers telephone support and a network conference every Thursday at 9 p.m. Eastern time for the first 150 callers. Check the website or call 877-232-2992 in advance to obtain a guest ID number. Also see www.askdrjamie.net.

Organizations Outside the U.S.

Alzheimer Society
www.alzheimer.ca/english/society/mission.htm

This Canadian organization provides information and education and referrals for support services.

Alzheimer Europe
www.alzheimer-europe.org

This website includes overviews and details on Alzheimer's care in European countries.

Alzheimer's Disease International
www.alz.co.uk

An umbrella organization for Alzheimer's associations around the world.

Caregiving

National Alliance for Caregiving
301-718-8444

www.caregiving.org

This nonprofit coalition of national organizations focused on family caregiving conducts research, provides information, and offers other resources.

National Center on Caregiving
800-445-8106; 415-434-3388

www.caregiver.org

This organization, which is part of the Family Caregiver Alliance, has programs in education, services, research, and advocacy and is the premier starting place. The website offers information, online discussion groups, and the Family Care Navigator, a state-by-state directory of programs, support, and services for caregivers and their loved ones (www.caregiver. org/caregiver/jsp/fcn_content_node.jsp?nodeid=2083).

U.S. Administration on Aging, Department of Health and Human Services
202-619-0724

www.aoa.gov

This federal agency offers many resources and services, including the Eldercare Locator (www.eldercare.gov; 800-677-1116), which helps older adults and their families and caregivers find information on senior services.

Lotsa Helping Hands
www.lotsahelpinghands.com

Free web-based service for organizing a loved one's family and community to provide assistance and support, and help with communication and sharing information.

Visiting Nurse Associations of America
202-384-1420
www.vnaa.org

The national association of nonprofit visiting nurse agencies and home healthcare providers, with the aim of offering cost-effective and compassionate home care. Check out your local chapter.

For Children and Teenagers

Alzheimer's Association
www.alz.org/living_with_alzheimers_just_for_kids_and_teens.asp

Information and helpful links for helping kids and teens understand Alzheimer's and connect with a loved one with the disease.

Mayo Foundation for Medical Education and Research
www.mayoclinic.com/health/alzheimers/HQ00216

A good resource for helping children understand Alzheimer's.

Additional Internet Resources

Alzheimer Research Forum
www.alzforum.org

A free forum with a great deal of research-based basic factual information about issues related to Alzheimer's.

Mayo Clinic
www.mayoclinic.com/health/alzheimers-disease/DS00161

Information and reprints on all aspects of Alzheimer's are available at this website.

Medline Plus

www.nlm.nih.gov/medlineplus/alzheimersdisease.html

This website, which is a service of the U.S. National Library of Medicine, offers numerous links to valuable information and the latest research findings.

Books

General Information

Coste, J. K. 2004. *Learning to Speak Alzheimer's.* New York: Houghton Mifflin. This helpful book describes a technique called "habitation" to use to communicate with early-stage Alzheimer's people.

Davies, H., and M. Jensen. 1998. *Alzheimer's: The Answers You Need.* Forest Knolls, CA: Elder Books. A great practical book for those in the early stages of Alzheimer's.

Kuln, D. 2003. *Alzheimer's Early Stages: First Steps of Family, Friends and Caregivers.* Alameda, CA: Hunter House. Medical information and personal stories.

Lokvig, J., and J. D. Becker. 2004. *Alzheimer's A to Z: A Quick Reference Guide.* Oakland, CA: New Harbinger Publications. A brief but thorough review of Alzheimer's and related issues.

Mace, N. L., and P. V. Rabins. 2006. *The 36-Hour Day,* 4th ed. New York: Warner Books; Baltimore, MD: The Johns-Hopkins University Press. A comprehensive book about Alzheimer's that's especially helpful for caregivers.

Robinson, A., B. Spencer, and L. White. 1989. *Understanding Difficult Behaviors: Some Practical Suggestions for Coping with Alzheimer's Disease and Related Illnesses.* Ypsilanti, MI: Eastern Michigan University. This concise but thorough guide may be available through your local Alzheimer's Association.

Strauss, C. 2001. *Talking to Alzheimer's: Simple Ways to Connect When You Visit with a Family Member or Friend.* Oakland, CA: New Harbinger Publications. This book provides information about initiating conversations.

People with Early Alzheimer's Tell Their Stories

Davis, R. 1979. *My Journey into Alzheimer's Disease.* Wheaton, IL: Tyndale House Publishers.

Henderson, C. 1998. *Partial View: An Alzheimer's Journal.* Dallas, TX: Southern Methodist University Press.

McGowan, D. 1994. *Living in the Labyrinth: A Personal Journey Through the Maze of Alzheimer's.* New York: Dell Publishing.

Raushi, T. 2001. *A View from Within: Living with Early Onset Alzheimer's.* Albany, NY: Alzheimer's Disease and Related Disorders Association. Available from the New York City chapter of the Alzheimer's Association: 646-744-2900; www.alznyc.org/store

Rose, L. 1996. *Show Me the Way to Go Home.* Forest Knolls, CA: Elder Books.

Caregiving

American Medical Association and A. Perry. 2001. *American Medical Association Guide to Home Caregiving*. New York: John-Wiley and Sons.

Bell, V., and D. Troxel. 2002. *A Dignified Life: The Best Friends Approach to Alzheimer's Care: A Guide for Family Caregivers*. Deerfield Beach, FL: Health Communications.

Callone, P. R., C. Kudlacek, B. C. Vasiloff, J. Manternach, and R. A. Brumback. 2006. *Alzheimer's Disease: The Dignity Within*. New York: Demos Medical Publishing. A touching approach, sponsored by a chapter of the Alzheimer's Association.

Callone, P. R., C. Kudlacek, B. C. Vasiloff, J. Manternach, D. Min, and R. A. Brumback. 2005. *A Caregiver's Guide to Alzheimer's Disease: 300 Tips for Making Life Easier*. New York: Demos Medical Publishing. An excellent resource, sponsored by a chapter of the Alzheimer's Association.

Castleman, M., D. Gallagher-Thompson, and M. Naythons. 1999. *There's Still a Person in There: The Complete Guide to Treating and Coping with Alzheimer's*. New York: Penguin Putnam.

Caregiver Stories

ABOUT COUPLES

Davidson, A. 1997. *Alzheimer's, a Love Story: One Year in My Husband's Journey*. Secaucus, NJ: Carol Publishing. Poignant account of the author's husband in early to mid stage Alzheimer's.

Davidson, A. 2006. *A Curious Kind of Widow: Loving a Man with Advanced Alzheimer's.* McKinleyville, CA: Fithian Press. A heart-wrenching account of the author's husband in the later stages of the disease.

ABOUT MOTHERS

Caldwell, M. 1995. *Gone Without a Trace.* Forest Knolls, CA: Elder Books.

Dyer, J. 1996. *In a Tangled Wood: An Alzheimer's Journey.* Dallas, TX: Southern Methodist University Press. A daughter's story of her mother's illness.

McLay, E., and E. P. Young. 2007. *Mom's OK, She Just Forgets: The Alzheimer Journey from Denial to Acceptance.* New York: Prometheus Books.

ABOUT FATHERS

McAndrews, L. 1990. *My Father Forgets.* Maple City, MI: Northern Publishing Company.

FOR MALE CAREGIVERS

Alzheimer's Association, Iowa Golden Chapter. 1992. *Male Caregivers Guidebook: Caring for Your Loved One with Alzheimer's at Home.* Des Moines, IO: Alzheimer's Association, Iowa Golden Chapter. 1200 Pleasant Street, Des Moines, IO 50309.

For Children

Fox, M. 1984. *Wilfred Gordon McDonald Partridge*. Brooklyn, NY: Kane/Miller Publishers. A terrific book for preschool children.

Shriver, M. (author), and S. Spielgel (illustrator). 2004. *What's Happening to Grandpa?* New York: Little Brown and Company and Warner Books. This book is excellent.

Cultural Differences and Caregiving

Yeo, G., and D. Gallagher-Thompson. 2006. *Ethnicity and the Dementias*. New York: Routledge Taylor and Francis Group.

Caregiving and Activities

Bazan-Salazar, E. C. 2005. *Alzheimer's Activities That Stimulate the Mind*. New York: McGraw-Hill.

Hellen, C. R. 1992. *Alzheimer's Disease: Activity Focused Care*. Boston: Butterworth-Heineman. Comprehensive analysis of disruptive behaviors, what they mean, and which activities will minimize problems. For professionals and caregivers.

Sheridan, C. 1987. *Failure-Free Activities for the Alzheimer Patient: A Guidebook for Caregivers*. San Francisco: Cottage Books.

Alzheimer's and Spirituality

American Academy of Family Physicians. 2001. Patient handout: Spirituality and health. Page 89 from an article by G. Anandarajah and E. Hight, "Spirituality and medical practice: Using the HOPE questions as a practical tool for spiritual assessment." Available at www.aafp.org/afp/20010101/89ph.html.

Shamy, E. 2003. *A Guide to the Spiritual Dimension of Care for People with Alzheimer's Disease and Related Dementia.* London and New York: Jessica Kingsley Publishers. This comprehensive book includes a guide for pastors.

A Note About Websites

In evaluating other sites you may have discovered on your own, here are some suggestions from Bill Reiter, education coordinator, and Kathleen Kelly and Leah Ashkenazi of the Family Caregiver Alliance:

1. Who sponsors the site?

2. Is the information updated? Do outside experts review the information if the website isn't well-known?

3. What is the purpose of the site originator? Does it cost to become a member?

References

Aguglia, E., M. L. Onor, M. Trevisiol, C. Negro, M. Saina, and E. Maso. 2004. Stress in the caregivers of Alzheimer's patients: An experimental investigation in Italy. *American Journal of Alzheimer's Disease and Other Dementias* 19(4):248-252.

Akhondzadeh, S., and S. Abbasi. 2006. Herbal medicine in the treatment of Alzheimer's disease. *American Journal of Alzheimer's Disease and Other Dementias* 21(2):113-118.

Alzheimer's Association. 2007. *2007 Alzheimer's Disease Facts and Figures.* Chicago, IL.

———. 2009. *2009 Alzheimer's Disease Facts and Figures.* Chicago, IL.

American Journal of Alzheimer's Disease and Other Dementias. 2006. Newsbriefs: Music as therapy may ward off Alzheimer's disease. *American Journal of Alzheimer's Disease and Other Dementias* 21(2):79.

American Psychiatric Association (APA). 1994. *The Diagnostic and Statistical Manual of Mental Disorders* (DSM IV). Washington, DC: American Psychiatric Association.

Anandarajah, G., and E. Hight. 2001. Spirituality and medical practice: Using the HOPE questions as a practical tool for spiritual assessment. *American Family Physician* 63(1): 81-89.

Ancoli-Israel, S. 2004. Sleep disorders: Normal aging and dementia. Paper presented at the 6th Annual Update on Dementia: Translating Research into Practice. Stanford University School of Medicine. June 16, Palo Alto, California.

Arkin, S. M. 1998. Alzheimer memory training: Positive results replicated. *American Journal of Alzheimer's Disease and Other Dementias* 13(2):102-104.

———. 2000a. Alzheimer memory training: Students replicate learning successes. *American Journal of Alzheimer's Disease and Other Dementias* 15(3):152-162.

———. 2000b. Alzheimer memory training: Students replicate successes. Addendum on long-term retention. *American Journal of Alzheimer's Disease and Other Dementias* 15(5):314-315.

———. 2003. Student-led exercise sessions yield significant fitness gains for Alzheimer's patients. *American Journal of Alzheimer's Disease and Other Dementias* 18(3):159-170.

———. 2007. Language-enriched exercise plus socialization slows cognitive decline in Alzheimer's. *American Journal of Alzheimer's Disease and Other Dementias* 22(1):62-67.

Arkin, S. M., and N. Mahendra. 2001. Insight in Alzheimer's patients: Results of a longitudinal study using three assessment methods. *American Journal of Alzheimer's Disease and Other Dementias* 16(4):211-224.

Borysenko, J. 2008. Integrating science and spirit in end-of-life and bereavement care. Paper presented at the conference

Good Grief: The Heart of Healing. Menlo Park, California, sponsored by Kara Foundation, May 19.

Boss, P. *Ambiguous Loss*. 1999. Cambridge, MA: Harvard University Press.

Brody, J. E. 2008. Caring for family, caring for yourself. *New York Times*, November 18, section D, p. 7.

Buckley, C. 2009. All-night care for dementia's restless minds. *New York Times*, June 14, section MB, p. 1.

Carey, B. 2008a. For the brain, remembering is like reliving. *New York Times*, September 5, section A, p. 1.

————. 2008b. H. M., whose loss of memory made him unforgettable, dies. *New York Times*, December 5, section A, p. 1.

Cawthorn, A. 1995. A review of the literature surrounding the research into aromatherapy. *Complementary Therapies in Nursing and Midwifery* 1(4):118-120.

Clair, A. A. 2002. The effects of music therapy on engagement in family caregiver and care receiver couples with dementia. *American Journal of Alzheimer's Disease and Other Dementias* 17(5):286-290.

Clair, A. A., M. Matthews, and K. Kosloski. 2005. Assessment of active music participation as an indication for subsequent music making engagement for persons with midstage dementia. *American Journal of Alzheimer's Disease and Other Dementias* 20(1):37-40.

Clare, L. 2003. Managing threats to self: Awareness in early stage Alzheimer's disease. *Social Science Medicine* 57(6):1017-1029.

Cohen-Mansfield, J. C. 2001. Nonpharmacologic interventions for inappropriate behaviors in dementia. *American Journal of Geriatric Psychiatry* 9(4):361-381.

Cummings, J. L., and G. Cole. 2002. Alzheimer's disease. *Journal of the American Medical Association* 287(18):2335-2338.

Dempsey, M., and S. Baago. 1998. Latent grief: The unique and hidden grief of carers of loved ones with dementia. *American Journal of Alzheimer's Disease and Other Dementias* 13(2):84-91.

Dick, M. B. 1992. Motor and procedural memory in Alzheimer's disease. In *Memory Functioning in Dementia,* edited by L. Backman. North-Holland, the Netherlands: Elsevier Publishers.

Dollinger, S. C., K. Chwalisz, and E. O. Zerth. 2006. Tele-Help Line for Caregivers (TLC): A comprehensive telehealth intervention for rural family caregivers. *Clinical Gerontologist* 30(2):51-64.

Dowling, G. A. 1996. Behavior intervention strategies for sleep-activity disruption. *International Psychogeriatrics* 8(1):77-85.

Edelson, J. S., and W. H. Lyons. 1985. *Institutional Care of the Mentally Impaired Elderly.* New York: Van Nostrand Reinhold Company.

Fischer, C., R. Bozanovic-Sosic, and M. Norris. 2004. Review of delusions in dementia. *American Journal of Alzheimer's Disease and Other Dementias* 19(1):19-23.

Fleming, K. S., H. Kim, M. Doo, G. Maguire, and S. G. Potkin. 2003. Memory for emotional stimuli in patients with Alzheimer's disease. *American Journal of Alzheimer's Disease and Other Dementias* 18(6):340-342.

Foley, J. 1992. The experience of being demented. In *Dementia and Aging: Ethics, Values, and Policy Choices,* edited by R. H. Binstock, S. G. Post, and P. J. Whitehouse. Baltimore, MD: Johns Hopkins University Press.

Gallagher-Thompson, D., W. Haley, G. DeLois, M. Rupert, T. Argüelles, L. McKenzie Zeiss, C. Long, S. Tennestedt, and M. Ory. 2003. Tailoring psychological interventions for ethnically diverse dementia caregivers. *Clinical Psychology: Science and Practice* 10(4):423-438.

Gaugler, J. E., K. A. Anderson, C. R. Leach, C. D. E. Smith, F. A. Schmitt, and M. Mendiondo. 2004. The emotional ramifications of unmet need in dementia caregiving. *American Journal of Alzheimer's Disease and Other Dementias* 19(6):369-380.

Gentry, R. A., and J. E. Fisher. 2007. Facilitating conversation in elderly persons with Alzheimer's disease. *Clinical Gerontologist* 31(2):77-98.

Gerritsen, D. L., T. P. Ettema, E. Boelens, J. Bos, F. Hoogeveen, J. de Lange, L. Meihuizen, C. M. Scholzel-Dorenbos, and R. M. Droes. 2007. Quality of life in dementia: Do professional caregivers focus on the significant domains? *American Journal of Alzheimer's Disease and Other Dementias* 22(3):176-183.

Glick, T. H., and A. E. Dudson. 2005. Education and communication about memory: Using terminology of cognitive neuroscience. *American Journal of Alzheimer's Disease and Other Dementias* 20(3):141-143.

Harrison, B. E., G. R. Son, J. Kim, and A. L. Whall. 2007. Preserved implicit memory in dementia: A potential model for care. *American Journal of Alzheimer's Disease and Other Dementias* 22(4):286-293.

Hochhalter, A. K., A. B. Stevens, and O. Okonkwo. 2007. Structured practice: A memory intervention for persons with dementia. *American Journal of Alzheimer's Disease and Other Dementias* 21(6):424-430.

Holst, G., and I. R. Hallberg. 2003. Exploring the meaning of everyday life, for those suffering from dementia. *American*

Journal of Alzheimer's Disease and Other Dementias 18(6):359-365.

Jin, K., V. Galvan, L. Xie, X. O. Mao, O. F. Gorostiza, D. E. Bredsesen, and D. Greenberg. 2004a. Enhanced neurogenesis in Alzheimer's disease transgenic (PDGF-APP Sw, Ind) mice. *The National Academy of Sciences* 101(36):13363-13367.

Jin, K., A. Peel, X. O. Mao, L. Xie, B. Cottrell, and D. A. Greenberg. 2004b. Increased hippocampal neurogenesis in Alzheimer's disease. *Proceedings of the National Academy of Sciences*, 101:343-347.

Judge, K. S., C. J. Camp, and S. Orsulic-Jeras. 2000. Use of Montessori-based activities with dementia in adult day care: Effects on engagement. *American Journal of Alzheimer's Disease and Other Dementias* 15(1):42-46.

Kanter, L. 2008. Alzheimer's, memory and dementia. Paper presented at the Institute for Natural Resources, May 1, Palo Alto, CA.

Kennedy, R. 2005. The Pablo Picasso Alzheimer's therapy. *New York Times*, October 30, national edition, arts section, p. 1.

King, A. C., K. Baumann, P. O'Sullivan, S. Wilcox, and C. Castro. 2002. Effects of moderate-intensity exercise on physiological, behavioral, and emotional responses to family caregiving. *Journals of Gerontology: Series A, Biological Sciences and Medical Sciences* 57(1):M26-36.

Kosloski, K., and R. J. Montgomery. 1995. The impact of respite use on nursing home placement. *Gerontologist* 35(1):67-74.

LeDoux, J. E. 1993. Emotional memory systems in the brain. *Behavioural Brain Research* 58(1-2):69-79.

Leland, J. 2008. More men take the lead role in caring for elderly parents. *New York Times*, November 29, section A, p. 1.

Lewis, M. L., K. Hepburn, S. Narayan, and L. N. Kirk. 2005. Relationship matters in dementia caregiving. *American Journal of Alzheimer's Disease and Other Dementias* 20(6):341-348.

Lichtenberg, P. 2006. Assisting urban caregivers after nursing home placement: Results from two programs. *Clinical Gerontologist* 30(2):65-78.

Logsdon, R., S. M. McCurry, and L. Teri. 2006. Time-limited support groups for individuals with early stage dementia and their care partners: Preliminary outcomes from a controlled clinical trial. *Clinical Gerontologist* 30(2):5-19.

Mace, N. L., and P. V. Rabins. 2006. *The 36-Hour Day*, 4th ed. New York: Warner Books; Baltimore, MD: The Johns-Hopkins University Press.

Marseille, D. M., and D. H. S. Silverman. 2006. Recognition and treatment of Alzheimer's disease: A case-based review. *American Journal of Alzheimer's Disease and Other Dementias* 21(2):119-125.

Matteau, E., P. Landreville, L. Laplante, and C. Laplante. 2003. Disruptive vocalizations: A means to communicate in dementia? *American Journal of Alzheimer's Disease and Other Dementias* 18(3):147-153.

Mitchell, D. B. 1988. Memory and language deficits in Alzheimer's disease. In *Caring for the Alzheimer Patient*, edited by R. L. Dippel and J. T. Hutton. Buffalo, NY: Prometheus Books.

Montgomery, R. J. V., and K. D. Kosloski. 2002. Family caregiving: Change, continuity and diversity. In *Interventions in Dementia Care*, edited by P. Lawton and R. Rubenstein. New York: Springer Publishing Company.

Morris, R. G., and M. D. Kopelman. 1986. The memory deficits in Alzheimer-type dementia: A review. *Quarterly Journal of Experimental Psychology A* 38(4):575-602.

Onor, M. L., M. Trevisol, C. Negro, and E. Aguglia. 2007. Impact of multimodal rehabilitative intervention on demented patients and their caregivers. *American Journal of Alzheimer's Disease and Other Dementias* 22(4):261-272.

Ostwald, S. K., W. Duggleby, and K. W. Hepburn. 2002. The stress of dementia: View from the inside. *American Journal of Alzheimer's Disease and Other Dementias* 17(5):303-312.

Pearlin, L. L., T. Mullan, S. J. Semple, and M. M. Skaff. 1990. Caregiving and the stress process: An overview of concepts and their measures. *Gerontologist* 30(5):583-594.

Petersen, R. C. 2007. Mild cognitive impairment. *Continuum Lifelong Learning Neurology* 13(2):15-18.

———. 2008. Mild cognitive impairment: The current status. Presentation at 10th Annual Updates on Dementia: Translating Research into Practice, June 4, Palo Alto, CA.

Richeson, N. E. 2003. Effects of animal-assisted therapy on agitated behaviors and social interactions of older adults with dementia. *American Journal of Alzheimer's Disease and Other Dementias* 18(6):353-358.

Rikkert, M. G., J. P. Teunisse, and M. Vernooij-Dassen. 2005. One hundred years of Alzheimer's disease and the neglected second lesson of Alois Alzheimer on multicausality in dementia. *American Journal of Alzheimer's Disease and Other Dementias* 20(5):269-272.

Sabat, S. R. 2006. Implicit memory and people with Alzheimer's disease: Implications for caregiving. *American Journal of Alzheimer's Disease and Other Dementias* 21(1):11-14.

Sacks, O. 1987. *The Man Who Mistook His Wife for a Hat*. New York: Harper & Row.

Schneider, L. S., P. N. Tariot, K. S. Dagerman, S. M. Davis, J. K. Hsiao, M. S. Ismail, B. D. Lebowitz, C. G. Lyketsos, J. M.

Ryan, T. S. Stroup, D. L. Suttzer, D. Weintraub, and J. A. Lieberman. 2006. Effectiveness of atypical antipsychotic drugs in patients with Alzheimer's disease. *New England Journal of Medicine* 355(15):1525-1606.

Shimamura, A. P. 1986. Priming effects of amnesia: Evidence for a dissociable memory function. *Quarterly Journal of Experimental Psychology. A, Human Experimental Psychology.* 38(4):619-644.

Sink, K. M., K. F. Holden, and K. Yaffe. 2005. Pharmacological treatment of neuropsychiatric symptoms of dementia: A review of the evidence. *Journal of the American Medical Association* 293(5):596-608.

Small, J. A., J. Perry, and J. Lewis. 2005. Perceptions of family caregivers' psychosocial behavior when communicating with spouses who have Alzheimer's disease. *American Journal of Alzheimer's Disease and Other Dementias* 20(5):281-289.

Smith, D. H. 1992. Seeing and knowing dementia. In *Dementia and Aging: Ethics, Values, and Policy Choices*, edited by R. H. Binstock, S. G. Post, and P. J. Whitehouse. Baltimore, MD: Johns Hopkins University Press.

Spira, A. P., S. A. Beaudreau, D. Jimenez, M. A. Kierod, M. M. Cusing, H. L. Gray, and D. Gallagher-Thompson. 2007. Experiential avoidance, acceptance, and depression in dementia family caregivers. *Clinical Gerontologist* 30(4):55-64.

Talerico, K. A., L. K. Evans, and N. E. Strumpf. 2002. Mental health correlates of aggression in nursing home residents with dementia. *Gerontologist* 42(2):169-177.

Tannen, D. 1990. *You Just Don't Understand: Men and Women in Conversation.* New York: Morrow.

Taylor, J. L., L. Friedman, L. J. Sheikh, and J. A. Yesavage. 1997. Assessment and management of "sundowning phenomena." *Seminars in Clinical Neuropsychiatry* 2(2):113-122.

Teri, L., L. E. Ferretti, L. E. Gibbons, R. G. Logsdon, S. M. McCurry, W. A. Kukull, W. C. McCormick, J. D. Brown, and E. B. Larson. 1999. Anxiety in Alzheimer's disease: Prevalence and comorbidity. *Journals of Gerontology. Series A, Biological Sciences and Medical Sciences* 54(7):M348-352.

Teri, L., L. E. Gibbons, S. M. McCurry, R. Logsdon, D. M. Buchner, W. E. Barlow, A. Z. LaCroix, W. McCormick, and E. B. Larson. 2003. Exercise plus behavioral management in patients with Alzheimer disease. *Journal of the American Medical Association* 290(15):2015-2022.

Tucker, M. A., and W. Fishbein. 2008. Enhancement of declarative memory performance following a daytime nap is contingent on strength of initial task acquisition. *Sleep* 31(2): 197-203.

Wang, S. 2008. When Alzheimer's hits at 40. *Wall Street Journal,* November 14, section A, p. 1.

Whall, A. L., M. Balack, C. Groh, D. Yankou, B. Kupferschmid, and N. Foster. 1997. The effect of natural environments upon agitation and aggression in late-stage dementia. *American Journal of Alzheimer's Disease and Other Dementias* 12(5):216-220.

Worwood, S. E., and V. A. Worwood. 2003. *Essential Aromatherapy: A Pocket Guide to Essential Oils and Aromatherapy.* Novato, CA: New World Library.